Ageing and how to avoid it

By
Lynne D M Noble

Copyright 2023 Lynne D M Noble

Independently published

Contents

Dedication

This book is dedicated to all who wish to age successfully

Acknowledgement

Many thanks to all my friends who have supplied the inspiration to write this book.

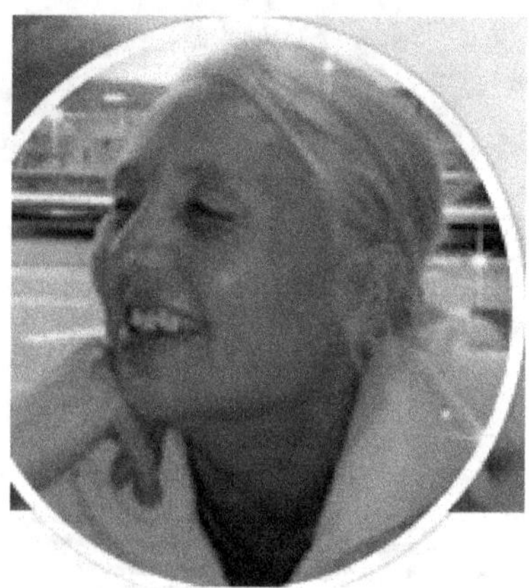

Including Laraine above aged 66 years.

Preface

The World Health Organisation defines health aging as the

Process of developing and maintaining the functional ability that enables wellbeing in older age.

Functional ability is about having the capabilities that enable all people to be and do what they have reason to value. This includes the person's ability to:

- Meet their basic needs
- Learn, grow and make decisions
- To be mobile
- To build and maintain relationships and
- To contribute to society

There isn't a *typical* older person. My mother and her four sisters are in their late eighties up to their mid-nineties and enjoy their independence greatly. They do not ail much at all and eat what they like. Some people appear to be physically and mentally older when they are in fifties. They appear to have slotted themselves into their own idea of how they believe older age should be.

When I was a child, I used to observe the ladies in their fifties and sixties. I was a curious child and I wanted to know why these ladies all cut their hair short and had a perm and a blue rinse. Most of them walked with the aid of a walking stick and complained of arthritic pains. They bemoaned their thinning hair. This did not go unnoticed by me. Up until then, I thought it was just men that went bald. In short, the individuality that these middle-aged ladies will have had when they were younger, had disappeared. They were like clones of each other. Sometimes I had difficulty knowing who was Mrs Smith and who was Mrs Brown; they all looked the same.

I also noticed that instead of walking smartly they began to wobble from side to side. This is an indication that balance is being affected but it doesn't have to happen. It really doesn't. A simple vitamin deficiency is well known to restore balance in a matter of days.

Hair tends to thin as you age so I am informed. There are lots of reasons why hair thins as you age and most can be corrected. I have spent too many hours looking at young people who have coloured their hair with harsh chemicals and wonder why their hair is falling out in clumps.

I have sat looking at elderly ladies having wisps of white hair being pulled into some sort of style to hide the pale pink scalp that is only too obvious. The brush that the hairdresser has used is full of thin soft strands of cotton wool hair. What happened to it?

Male pattern baldness is more difficult to treat but there are some simple things that can be undertaken to help slow the process down or restore some of the strands that have been lost.

Colour lost may be regained in some cases using some simple supplements or increasing these in the diet. In other cases, if a change of colour is desired than there are brands which are not harmful to the scalp. In some cases, you can make your own colours, shampoos and conditioners.

A couple of years ago when I was in the hairdressers, one of the clients sitting next to me was asked what she wanted doing with her hair. Without hesitation, she pointed at me and said, 'I want hair like that lady has got.'

Thick glossy hair is not the domain of the young. It is something that can be yours in your fifties and sixties or beyond.

It does not require HRT either although if it works for you then go for it.

My hair regime takes about 5 minutes plus washing time. I will share my secret with you.

Confidence is an attractive quality. Confident people are happy to develop their own personalities rather than try and emulate others. They develop a style which is unique and carry it with flair. They may be tall, they may be short, they may have curves or long slim limbs but they are happy in their own skin.

They are not slaves to fashion but look good equally in gardening gear or more formal dress. They do not fit into culturally acceptable boxes and it is often this uniqueness that draws others to them.

Of course, a large proportion of the differences in people of older age is - as WHO points out - due to the

Cumulative impact of advantage and disadvantage across people's lives.'

By the above it is referring to factors such as genes, our sex, ethnicity, level of education and financial resources.

Nevertheless, it does not take a great deal to start undoing the cumulative damage which disadvantage and neglect can bring in their wake. It certainly does not cost what the price of a shampoo, cut and set does nowadays.

A smooth, unlined skin and thick, glossy hair can continue to be yours as you age. Any aches and pains can be dealt with relatively easily. There is no need to slip into the mentality that older age is to be feared and that we have nothing to contribute to society. We have lived a lifetime, we have wisdom and the ability and confidence to change the things which need changing. We can grasp life with both hands and still look as good as those decades younger.

Every age group will have certain health challenges which appear specific to them. It would be unusual to find a childhood illness in the elderly but not in the young. We do not ignore the health conditions which appear peculiar to the young. If they need addressing, then they are addressed as best as time and resources allow. It should not be any difference in the older age group.

This book is intended to show you how to do just that.

What is Aging?

The Institute of Aging state that this phenomenon is associated with changes in a number or processes which include biological, physiological, psychological and social processes.

The actual causes of aging are not clear. Popular theories argue that it is an accumulation of damage which cause biological systems to fail. Examples of such damage are:

- Free radical theory
- Cross-linking theory
- Wear and tear

Other theories believe in the programmed aging concept where internal processes are programmed to run down eventually. This theory includes concepts such as:

- Immunological theory
- Senescence theory

We shall look at some of the theories in more detail later.

Some age related processes are benign. That is, they cause us no physical harm. One example of this is greying hair. Others changes can be harmful. There are for example:

- Decline in the activities of daily life
- Increasing frailty
- Increasing susceptibility to disease and disability
- Decline in the functions of senses

There is not one single explanation to account for the aging process. However, studies have shown that that while aging will occur, the rate at which it occurs can be slowed.

A study[1] took identical twin and looked at the differences in the physical appearance. Any differences found were thought to be due to environmental differences. The twins showing the greatest amount of differences in visible aging signs also had the greatest degree of discordance between personal lifestyle choices and habits.

The two main external factors accounting for this difference were

- Smoking
- Sun exposure

Other lifestyle factors which have the potential to increase the progression of aging are

- Stress
- Diet
- Exercise
- Medication
- Alcohol consumption

---

[1] https://www.ncbi.nlm.nih.gov/pubmed/10597816

Of course having longevity genes does help but in this study they found that the influences on aging may be highly overrated. It appears that lifestyle choices exert more effects on physical aging.

Middle age – what's that?

When I began this book, I had to define what middle age was. When I was much younger middle age was the time that was always ten years older than you were yourself.

This has all changed. An article in the Telegraph by Richard Alleyne, Science Correspondent, stated that according to a study, the average Briton believes that youth ends at 35 and old begins at 58. The years in between – 23 years – is apparently middle age.

This was news to me!

The Oxford English Dictionary defines middle age as being between the age of 45 and 65.

According to WHO most developed countries have accepted the chronological age of 65 years as a definition of 'elderly individuals. It appears to be associated with the age at which one can begin to receive pension benefits. This may change as countries such as the USA, Canada and the UK are raising the retirement age.

Elderly age can be categorised into three different groups:

Young old: 60-74 years' old

Old old: 75-84 years' old

Oldest old: > 85 years' old

We could also define our age using Intrinsic Capacity. This comprises

'All the mental and physical capacities that a person can draw on and includes their ability to walk, think, see, hear and remember.'

WHO

According to WHO the level of intrinsic capacity is influenced by a number of factors including the presence of diseases, injuries and age-related changes.

We can increase our intrinsic capacity because we can address many disease states and injuries as well as slow down the progression of many age related changes.

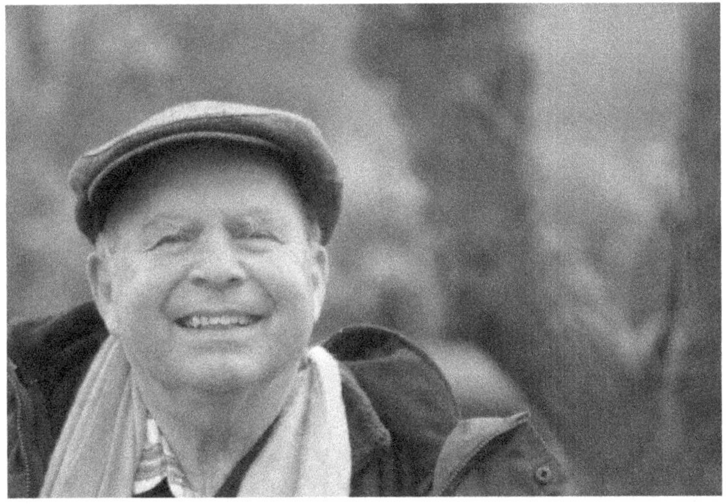

Michael (above) is seventy-four. He leads a full and busy life. He is still waiting for his first wrinkle! He does not have high blood pressure or heart disease or joint problems. He likes peanut butter and Marmite. He eats what he likes and doesn't pay much attention to the current wisdom of 'healthy' eating.

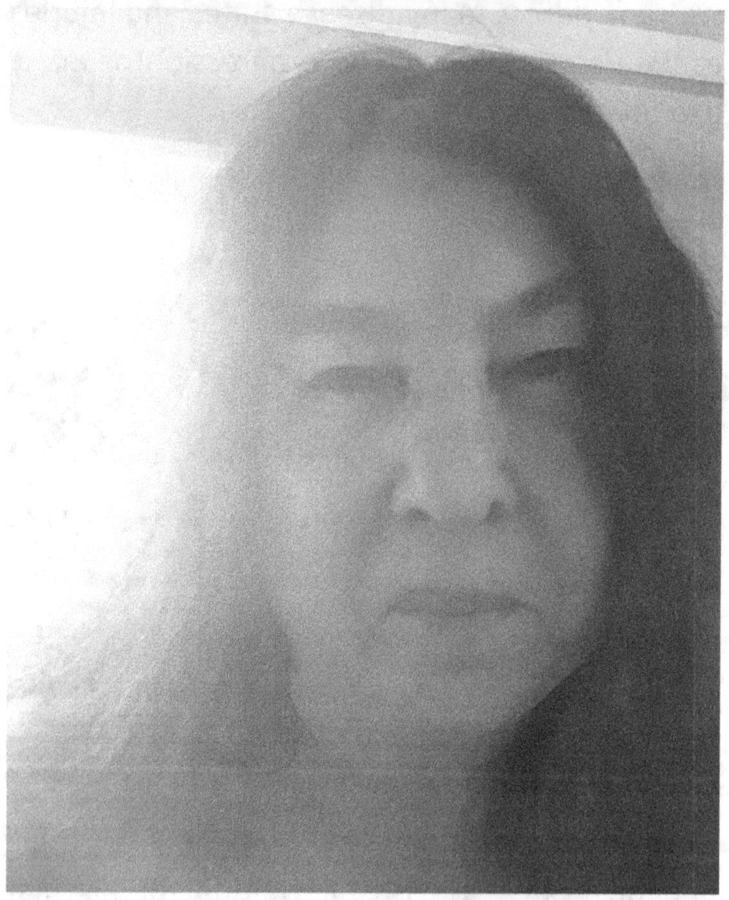

Author Lynne Noble aged 68 years.

When you talk to people who have aged successfully, one of the recurring themes is that they are not slaves to the latest diet fads. They tend to eat what they like and not what is the latest idea of 'healthy.'

However, their diets do appear to be higher in fat and lower in sugar. Further, none of them smoke. A diet higher in fat and lower in simple carbohydrates is extremely vital for a smooth unlined skin and good health. We shall examine this concept in the next chapter.

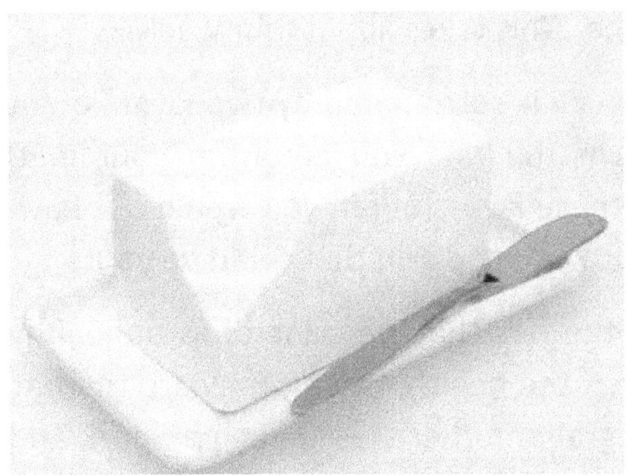

Healthy fats and nutrients for healthy skin

When I look at people who are on very low fat diets, their skin does not look smooth and unlined or particularly healthy. This does not mean that salad does not have some health benefits, it does. It is just that it does not help form smooth, unlined skin. That is the domain of healthy fats.

The outer layers of your skin were originally created much further down in the dermis. They are pushed up, layer by layer, until they reach the surface. This takes about four weeks.

Each skin cell is surrounded by two layers of fat made from the fats you eat from your diet. Without these layers of fat, you would not have the smooth, unlined skin that could be yours.

Many of the fats that we think of as unhealthy are, in fact, the healthy ones. They are the fats that our grandmother's used such as pork and beef dripping, lard and butter. These – and the fats found in oily fish – are the fats which give us a soft glowing skin. They do not cause inflammation in the way that the vegetable oils such as sunflower and rapeseed oil do. These animal fats do not produce free radicals when used in cooking since their smoking temperature is much higher than that of vegetable oils and margarine. Free radicals are aging. They do not promote youthful skin.

Lard is used in many cosmetics nowadays as it moisturises beautifully and, as it is similar to our skin, tends not to produce any allergy.

Lard also has the advantage of containing lots of vitamin D. This is a regulatory vitamin (it helps keep the immune system working as it should) which is responsible for many actions in your body necessary for good health.

At this point some of you may be saying that saturated fat is bad for your cholesterol levels. This isn't true either. Saturated fat actually helps change the small dense LDL into the larger, fluffier, more benign type. Lard and dripping and butter are good for you and have the added benefit of tasting better, too.

LDL has been found to be associated with longevity and good cognitive function. LDL helps neutralise bacterial toxins so that they do not damage tissue. LDL helps synthesise vitamin D from the sun's rays and it helps form bile salts which are necessary to emulsify dietary fat so that the vitamins ADEK – which are vital for health - can be absorbed.

The best way to discover how good these saturated fats are for your skin is to ditch all the vegetable oils and margarine and, take a picture of your skin as it is now. Then go to the supermarket, buy butter, cream, eggs, dripping and lard and use those for cooking and eating. Take a picture 5 weeks later. You will notice the difference.   Your skin should be soft and blooming – just how it used to be when you were much younger.

I expect that the next objection raised about eating saturated fat will be that fat will increase body mass. This is also not true. In order to lay down fat in your body you need to raise insulin levels. Fat does not raise insulin levels. It is sugar which raises insulin levels and when these are raised they store the extra energy, known as triglycerides, in fat cells.

You do not need sugar for energy. Fat can also produce energy in a process called ketosis. There are some amino acids – the building blocks of protein – such as glutamine which can also be used directly by cells as a source of energy.

The Atkins diet which was based on protein and fat -and little or no carbohydrate - was found to be one of the healthiest diets that there were. Those on the Atkins diet still lost weight, even though they were eating far more fat. Their waistlines reduced, their blood pressure and cholesterol levels decreased. All in all, they were far healthier on the high fat diet than they ever were on a diet full of simple carbohydrates found in cakes, sugar and biscuits, sweets and anything with added sugar.

The omega 3 fats found in oily fish not only form the skin cell membrane structure but they - unlike the omega 6 fats - are anti-inflammatory in nature.   Mild, chronic inflammation, may not appear red and angry but subclinical inflammation retains fluid in the cells so that the neat smooth lines associated with the facial features of those much younger - and which give a more youthful appearance – are lost.

In addition, omega 3 suppresses a hormone produced by the liver called insulin-like growth factor.   This hormone can reduce spots and blemishes.

Unfortunately, the amount of omega 6 fat that we have in our diet, borders on dangerous levels. It is not surprising that the amount of inflammatory diseases has risen with the advent of pro-inflammatory vegetable oils and margarines containing trans-fats.   Now trans-fats have been taken out of margarine.   They were a risk factor for all sorts of disease.

Margarine may have been made slightly healthier but it is still not healthy.

These best thing we can do with such oils is place them in the bin for disposal.

People who are on low fat diets will also have thinning hair which will break easily. Good hair comes from the inside. Hair needs good dietary fats. We shall turn to the subject of healthy hair later.

Fat soluble vitamins

Low fat diets do not provide us with enough fat soluble vitamins which have a number of health giving benefits. The fat soluble vitamins are ADEK.

Vitamin A

Vitamin A encourages healthy skin cell production and it also helps stimulate fibroblasts. Fibroblasts are responsible for making collagen and producing the framework for tissues that keep skin firm and healthy. They also play a critical role in wound healing.

There are two main forms of vitamin A – retinoids and carotenoids. Both types are converted to retinol by your liver. It is either stored there or transported by the lymphatic system to cells throughout the body

Retinoids are able to be absorbed by the skin very well. They stimulate production of new skin cells. The topical Retinol A was prescribed to people with fine lines and wrinkles and worked very well to smooth out skin out making it look much younger.

Without retinol our skin can become very dry. A deficiency of this can cause a condition which plugs up your hair follicles leading to raised papules on the skin.

Carotenoids are high in anti-oxidants. Research published in the European Journal of Pharmaceutics and Biopharmaceutics stated that a diet high in carotenoids such as beta carotene can prevent premature skin aging, skin diseases and cell damage. [2]

---

[2] https://www.ncbi.nlm.nih.gov/pubmed/23246796

Retinoids can be found in animal products such as:

- Salmon
- Beef liver
- Dairy products
- Eggs
- Oily fish

Carotenoids can be found in plant products such as:

- Carrots
- Tomatoes
- Sweet potatoes
- Leafy green vegetables
- Fruits such as mangoes, plums and apricots

Too much carotenoid in the diet can cause the skin to turn yellow or orange but, once the amount of carotenoids is reduced, this discolouration disappears.

Vitamin D

Vitamin D is another vital substance which modifies the aging process. It helps to influence longevity and impacts on many processes with are associated with age-related disease. Studies showed that vitamin D engaged with longevity genes and extended lifespan by 33%.

How does vitamin D extend lifespan? Proteins have to keep their shape if they are to function properly but as aging progresses, this is less likely to happen. This leads to an accumulation of toxic, misfolded proteins which are found in a number of conditions such as Alzheimer's disease.

 Misfolded proteins are also found in type 2 diabetes.

Vitamin D2, which is converted into the active form of vitamin D – vitamin D3 - suppressed protein insolubility in worm studies. This prevented the toxicity caused by beta-amyloid protein which is a misfolded protein associated with Alzheimer's disease.   As such vitamin D has the potential to prolong lifespan.

Nearly every cell in the body has receptors for vitamin D which shows just how important it is for the overall health of the body.

Older people are particularly susceptible to vitamin D deficiency. They are less likely to absorb it from their diet. Further, the skin becomes less able to manufacture vitamin D from the sun's rays.

Cholesterol is needed to manufacture vitamin D from the sun's rays so the mass medication of individual's with statins, which lowers cholesterol, is setting up them up for a deficiency state.

Current recommendations for older people, that is for those aged 55 years or older are 2000 IU's of vitamin D3 daily. This is probably too low since absorption of nutrients becomes less effective as we age. This may be partially due to a lack of fat in the diet. Fat is needed to help absorb fat soluble vitamins but currently the (erroneous) assumption is that very low fat or no fat diets are good for us.

Vitamin D is probably better taken in supplement form since it is just about impossible to get the recommended daily intake from diet.

Sources of Vitamin D

- Fatty fish like mackerel and salmon
- Fortified foods like some cereals, soy milk
- Beef liver
- Cheese
- Egg yolks

A study in *International Journal of Biomedical Science* has shown that vitamin D can be safely and effectively absorbed through the skin.

Some people open a cod liver oil capsule and apply it to their skin. This will provide both vitamin A and D. Both vitamins can be absorbed by the skin.

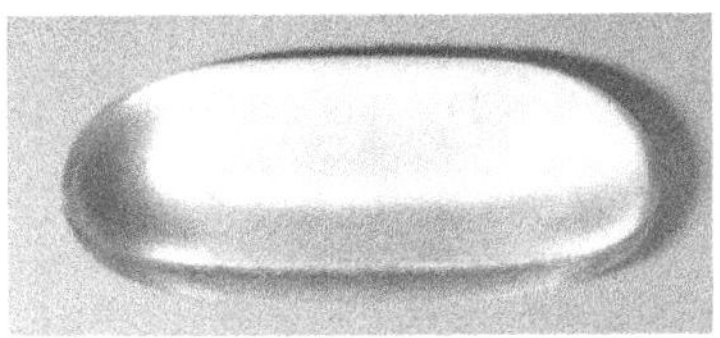

Vitamin D also produces its own antimicrobial proteins and so protects against many infections.

Vitamin E

The effect of the sun and its ability to damage skin is well known. Most of the visible aging of your skin – wrinkles, pigmentation, sun spots and reduced skin elasticity – are due to the ultra violet rays from the sun.

Current thinking is to use a high sun protection factor cream. However, these creams and oils often contain carcinogens. Further, the sun provides our vitamin D needs in the summer months so using a sun protection cream is counterproductive.

There are a number of nutrients which protect the skin from sun damage. Lycopene is a carotenoid which is found mainly in tomatoes although other red fruits, including water melons, also contain some useful lycopene.

How do tomatoes protect your skin? Well, the lycopene in them absorb both UVA and UVB rays so that the damaging effects are reduced.

Although lycopene exists in supplemental form, it is far better to obtain it in diet. It is not difficult to incorporate into pasta dishes or, if you prefer, a glass of tomato juice with a meal is not a hardship.

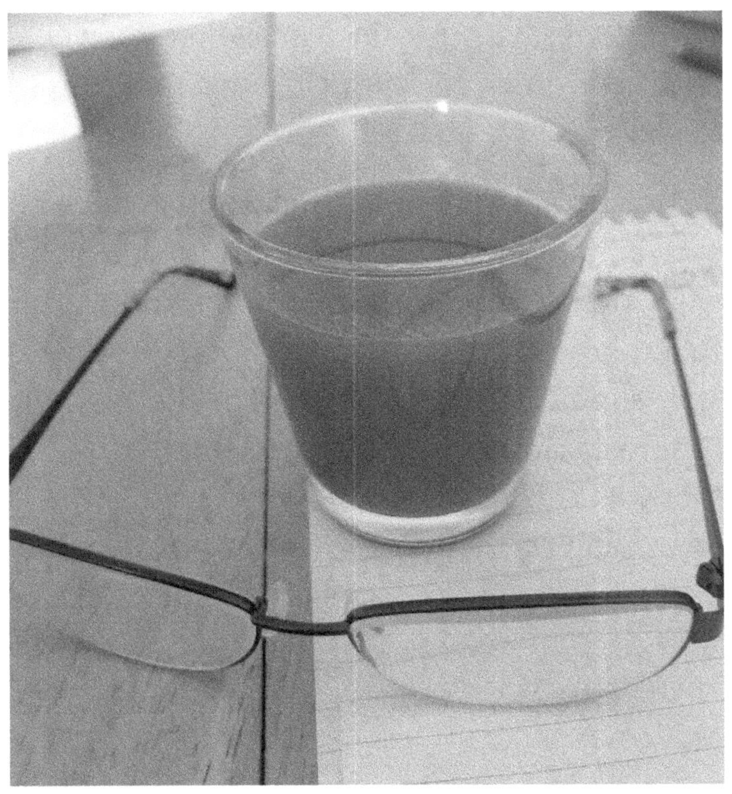

Tomato juice contains lycopene which has effective sun protection.

Astaxanthin has a remarkable reputation for protecting against UVB rays which cause sunburn in the outer layers of the skin. In addition, it can protect against the deeper layers being damaged by the UVA rays which are responsible for skin damage which would result in loss of elasticity and premature wrinkles.

If going abroad then supplementing with astaxanthin should be a priority if you don't wish to use a sun cream. However, for all year round protection then adding sockeye salmon, krill, shrimp, crab and lobster to the diet will raise astaxanthin levels.   It should be noted that wild caught sockeye salmon has four times more astaxanthin than the farmed variety.

There are also three antioxidants which have proven benefits in decreasing the effect of the sun on the skin and actually prevent further damage. These are

- Vitamin E
- Selenium
- Vitamin C

Antioxidants stop agents called free radicals from damaging cells in the skin and body.

Antioxidants are better taken in food as part of a healthy diet.

Vitamin E is a fat soluble nutrient and blood vessel dilator which increases the blood flow to tissues helping to bathe them in oxygen. Good sources of vitamin E are wheat germ and nuts and green leafy vegetables such as spinach and dark green cabbage.

The recommended daily amount of vitamin E is 15mg or 400 IU's daily.

Selenium has long been known to protect the skin from sun damage. Selenium carries this out through its role as a vital component of selenoproteins which help make DNA and protect against cell damage. In addition, selenium protects against toxic minerals and toxic substances made in the body and

Maintains healthy hair and skin

Protects the body as an antioxidant

Preserves normal liver function

Acts as an anti-inflammatory agent

Maintains healthy heart

All of which will impact on the health – and look – of the skin.

A deficiency is easily achieved if living off a diet of refined and processed foods. Further, foods grown on a selenium deficient soil increase that risk.

The recommended intake is no more than 200mcg from food.

Good food sources are;

Organ meats

Fish and shellfish

Muscle meats

Wholegrains

Cereals

Dairy products

Fruit and vegetables

Bearing in mind that for these foods to contain selenium they must be grown on selenium rich soil for direct consumption or for animals to eat to convert into animal products for our consumption.

By far the best source of selenium is found in brazil nuts where 2 brazil nuts will supply your daily recommended intake of selenium.

However, the main form of selenium to be found in peanuts, (when grown on selenium sufficient soil), is combined with the selenoproteins and forms a very high form of soluble protein found in this legume.

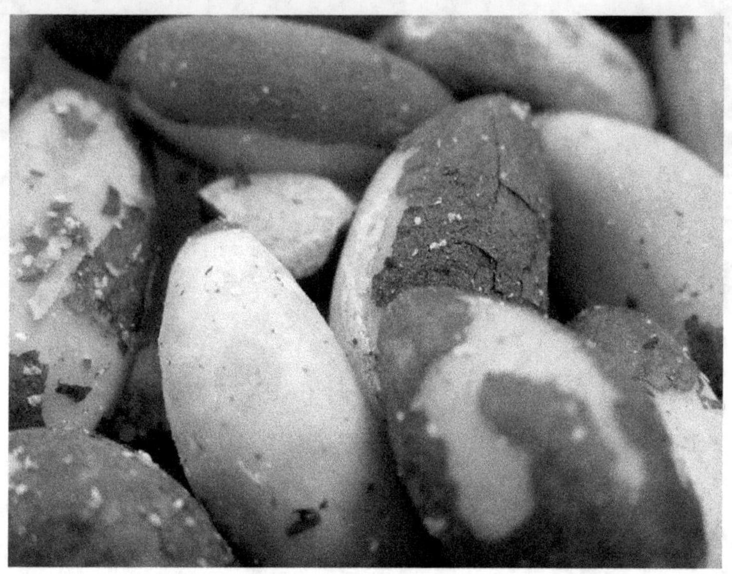

Two brazil nuts provide your total daily requirements of selenium.

Vitamin C - a water soluble vitamin - is a powerful antioxidant with superior anti-inflammatory properties. It helps to maintain collagen, helps resist infection, activates folic acid, is required for the synthesis of anti-stress hormones and is known as the antiscorbutic vitamin.

Scurvy is the deficiency caused by a vitamin C deficiency. Given the range of functions that vitamin C has and the dubious diets of many, it is quite likely that many people are suffering from sub clinical scurvy so what happens exactly with this condition?

Given its many important roles in the growth, development and healing of your skin and connective tissue, its role in strengthening blood vessels and absorbing iron – the former would lead to fragile vessels and very easy bruising – it is easy to see how a deficiency would age the skin rapidly.

Collagen is the major protein of connective tissue of which skin and bones, tendons and ligaments are composed. Connective tissue helps to give our facial features shape and support.

In addition, its role as an antioxidant helps protect cells against damage from free radicals. Free radicals are the products left over from normal cell metabolism and are injurious to health causing inflammation and, if it continues, damage which may not be reversible.

Vitamin C's ability to heal wounds is superior, helping to seal an unhealed wound within hours where it has remained unhealed without the support of extra vitamin C.

The recommended daily intake was set many years ago at an amount that was needed to avoid scurvy. This amount was set at 30mg but while it may prevent scurvy it does not address the needs of numerous functions in the body including the much higher requirements for good connective tissue health. When we look at respiratory health, we find that a whopping 6-8g acts therapeutically in cases of infections like pneumonia. With cancerous conditions, 60g or more of vitamin C has been given where bowel tolerance has not been reached, indicating how rapidly vitamin C has been used up before tissue saturation has occurred.

For those wondering what bowel tolerance is, it refers to the phenomenon that occurs when the tissues are saturated with vitamin C. Once saturation has been reached then the bowel releases its watery contents rapidly. The idea is to note the amount that indicates bowel tolerance and reduce that by 10% on a daily basis.

Fruit and vegetables are a good source of vitamin C but they have to be fresh. Vitamin C degrades rapidly in sunlight, with storage and will readily leach into water as it is a water soluble vitamin.

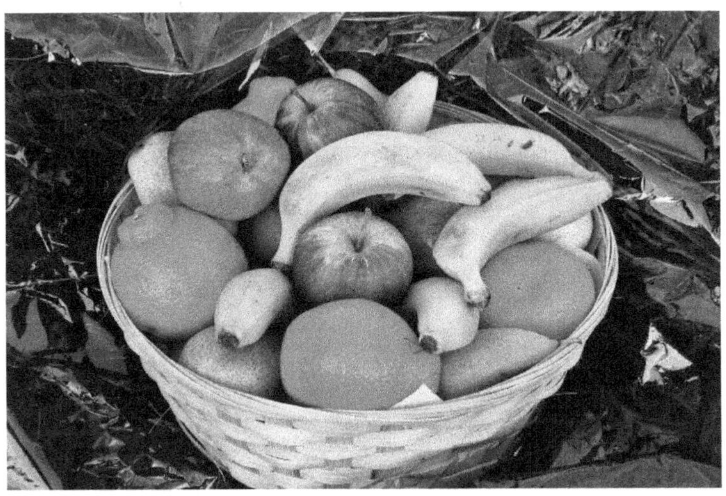

Fruit a great source of vitamin C

Vitamin K

This is a little known vitamin with huge benefits for the older person. Studies have shown that vitamin K is required to maintain skin elasticity. It is linked to fewer varicose veins. The production of a protein – MGP – which is crucial to the health of the vascular system, is dependent on this vitamin.

Without sufficient vitamin K calcification can affect the elastic fibres in the blood vessels, skin and eyes. The subsequent reduced blood flow can make the individual look less healthy as the flow of oxygen is reduced. The skin may take on a white or greyish pallor – which is very ageing - rather than the healthy pink colour acquainted with the young.

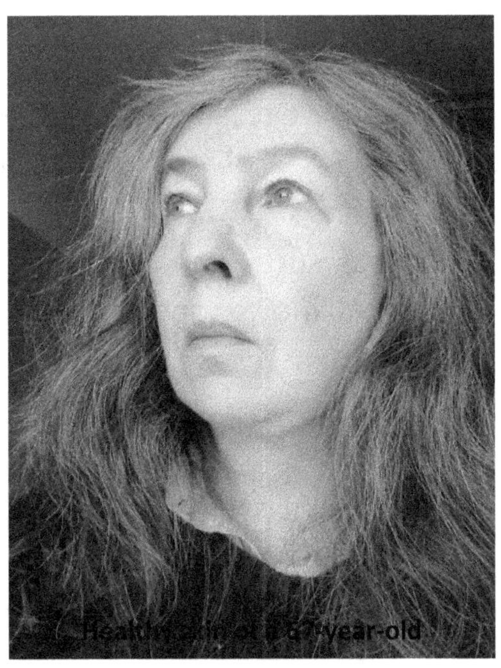

In addition, Vitamin K helps to stop your arteries from hardening. Further, it keeps calcium in your bones and not in your arteries. Thus it has a preventative role in heart disease.

Vitamin K2 is synthesised in the bowel but antibiotic therapy would reduce the amount made. In addition, vitamin K is found in:

- Green leafy vegetables – kale, spinach, turnip greens, collards, chard, parsley, green lettuce
- Vegetables such as Brussels sprouts, broccoli, cauliflower and cabbage
- Fish, liver, meat, eggs and cereals.

Eat foods containing vitamin K with a little fat – for example, butter – as vitamin K is fat soluble and needs the addition of a little dietary fat for it to be absorbed.

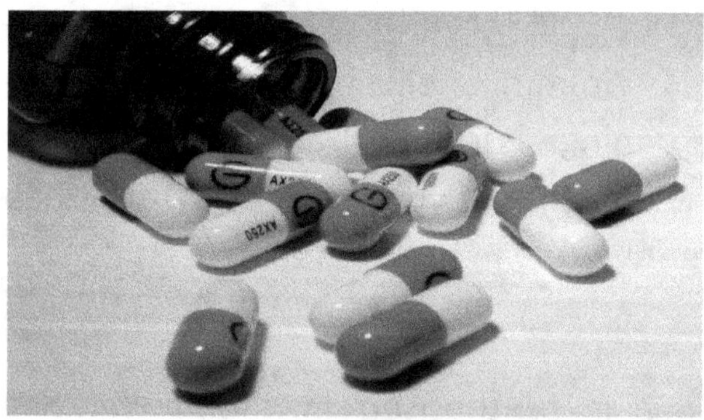

Antibiotics inhibit the synthesis of vitamin K in the gut

The Role of Sugar in speeding up the aging process.

Sugar is one of the most harmful substances we can ingest. The graph on the next page below shows the amount of sugar consumed in the UK

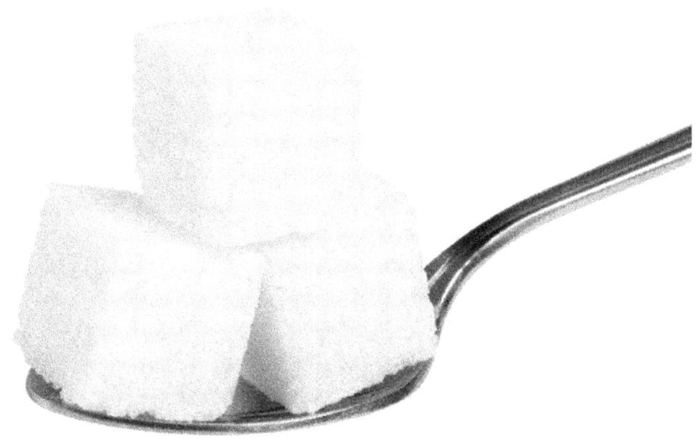

Sugar can cause rapid aging. Advanced Glycation End products (AGE's) are proteins or lipids that when exposed to sugar become glycated. Once attached they are referred to as being glycated and become proinflammatory molecules which initiate inflammation. They contribute to a state of atherosclerosis especially in diabetics where the AGE process is particularly troublesome due to the higher circulating sugars found in those with this condition.

Graph showing the association between sugar

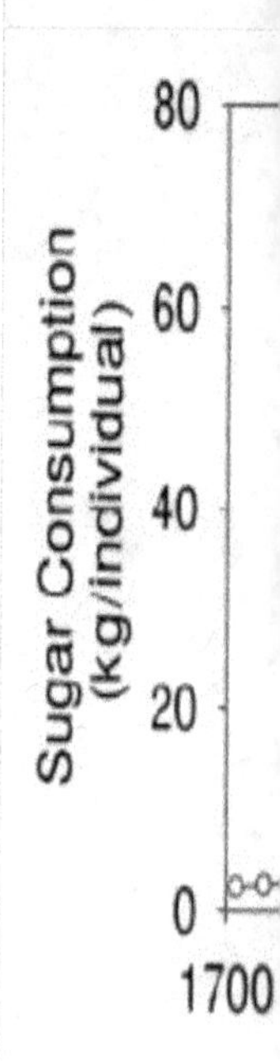

consumption and obesity between1700-1978.[3]

---

[3] [3] https://www.researchgate.net/figure/Sugar-intake-per-capita-in-the-United-Kingdom-from-1700-to-1978-30-31-E-and-in-the_fig1_5924426

As can be seen from the graph, sugar consumption is associated with obesity.

 Obesity is not all bad. It is a complex issue and the BMI charts that surgeries use do not actually measure the amount of fat that you have. They do not differentiate between those with lots of muscle mass which weighs more than fat. These charts were developed for an entirely different reason.[4]

In addition, there is enough research to show that older people live longer if they have more fat reserves. Part of this may be due to the fact that during prolonged illness, these extra energy reserves are invaluable. Indeed, as weight drops – if the patient does not feel like eating – the fat cells release vitamin D.

Vitamin D synthesises its own antimicrobial peptide called cathelicidin which has antiviral, antibacterial, antifungal and 'anti' everything else. The human body has, in effect, thought of everything in order to survive.

---

[4] See A Weighty Issue by Lynne D M Noble. For more information on this.

Being obese in a world which values 'thinness' can be damaging to confidence. In a recent survey I carried out with 20 men of different ages ranging from 18 years to 75 years, I asked what they thought was the most attractive feature in a woman. Their answers included:

A smile

A natural look – no make-up!

Proper curves

Intelligent eyes

Sensitivity

A calm nature

A personality

warmth

Not one mentioned they found slimness attractive. That doesn't mean to say that they don't but it was not at the top of their list of what they found attractive in a female. Physical characteristics were not as prized as personality.

My own thoughts are that our idea of attractiveness has been manipulated by those who would seek to profit from it. If society can be conned into believing that only slimness of the human form can be valued then there is a lot of money to be made from new-fangled slimming diets – generally promoted by celebrities - slimming aids such as protein powders, shakes and incredibly expensive calorie counted chocolate bars and soups. All the while the media condemn accusingly if the individual does not fit into a particular box.

These diets rarely provide the necessary nutrients for the synthesis of elastin and collagen.

Diets that are high in sugar can damage elastin and collagen in the skin. Elastin is a protein in connective tissue that allows tissues to resume their shape after stretching or contracting. Without this elasticity, skin sags and wrinkles.

Elastin is formed from smaller amino acids such as

- Glycine

- Proline

- Valine

- Alanine

We will return to these amino acids shortly.

Collagen is the most abundant protein in your body. It is a major component of connective tissues that make up tendons, skin and muscles for example. It provides you skin with structure and helps strengthen your bones.

Collagen boosting foods are:

- leafy greens

- vitamin C

- bone broth – this is an amazing source of collagen boosting nutrition as is any food that contains gelatine.

When sugar and protein or fat combine they produce something called Advanced Glycation End products. These can damage collagen and elastin producing sagging skin and wrinkles. They accelerate the effects of aging.

As collagen and elastin are renewed every four weeks there is the potential – if sugar is reduced dramatically in the diet – to produce much smoother and less wrinkled skin in that time scale.

The four amino acids required for younger looking skin

These are all small molecules

Glycine can be found in bone broth, wine gums, gummy bears, meat, fish and egg whites. Glycine also has the added benefit of enhancing sleep.

Valine is a branched chain amino acid. These help break down muscle tissue during exercise. It also helps the formation of structural proteins to avoid wrinkling and sagging.

Valine is found in cheese, soybeans, beef, lamb, chicken, pork, nuts, seeds, fish, beans, mushrooms and whole grains.

Proline is a major building block of skin and helps to keep its youthful appearance. Proline can break down protein to help create healthy cells and connective tissues. It helps promote a firmer skin especially when the major damage is sun related.

Alanine helps build lean muscle mass and helps improve physical functioning in the elderly.

Alanine is found in meats but it is also capable of being manufactured in the body.

Malic acid and skin health

Malic acid is one of a group of substances called alpha hydroxyl acids. These are capable of penetrating the skin to support collagen production which in turn helps maintain elasticity and suppleness.

Malic acid can decrease melanin which contribute to the age spots associated with older age. It appears in many expensive anti-aging skin care products.

Two fruits which are abundant in malic acid are apples and pears. These can be eaten or juiced to provide a cleanser since malic acid can be absorbed through the skin.

When you are eating an apple, cut off a sliver and rub it gently over any age spots.

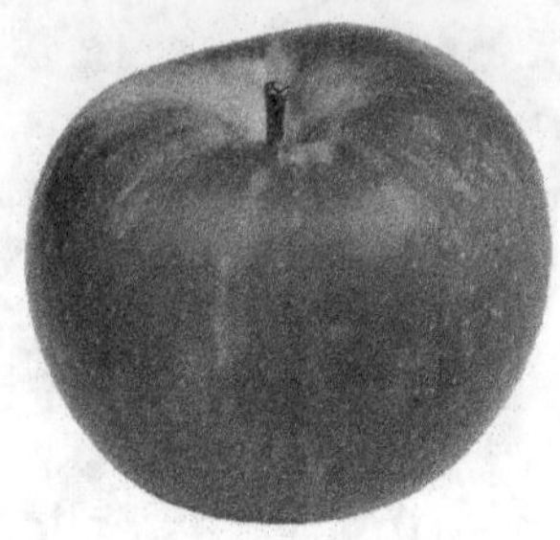

Malic acid is fairly mild but as it helps slough off the dead cells in the outer layers of the skin. It can help keep the complexion looking fresh.

Skin does not need washing with lotions and soap. Soap is slightly alkaline and skin prefers to be slightly acidic. The slight acidity helps to keep the skin protected from bacterial growth.

The best beauty routine is a flannel dipped in some warm water which is wiped over the face gently. If skin is very dry, then add a couple of drops of rosemary oil or castor oil to the water. The flannel is just rough enough to take the dead skin cells off the surface, in the same way that malic acid does, leaving a fresher complexion.

Some people dip the flannel in water, wring it out and put it in the microwave for 30 seconds. This has the added benefit of sterilising the flannel before use.

Some people develop very flaky skin on their legs as they age. Some of the flakiness may be due to a vitamin deficiency. One of the best moisturisers for this type of thing is to use warm castor oil. It plumps up and protects skin, from damage, quite quickly.

To help some of the fluid drain from the sinuses and facial tissues which will take away any puffiness, find the hollow just behind your ear lobe and *gently* stretch the skin. Do this three times on both sides of the ear. You should be able to feel the sinuses drain into the back of the throat.

Under your ear, starting from your jaw line pull the skin down gently again, three times on both sides.

Finally, stroke down your nose three times each side. The strokes have to be very light. If you are heavy handed, the tissue will react by drawing more fluid in.

This form of lymphatic drainage can take a few years off you.

Hair Growth and Health

They say that a good head of hair is a woman's crowning glory but it is also a man's too. Strong glossy hair is not just for the young. In most cases a good head of hair can be kept until very old age provided harsh chemicals are not used. Males, of course, have a disadvantageous as they are prone to male pattern baldness. If this is treated early enough there is a good chance that hair loss will be delayed.

The hair follicle goes through three stages:

Anagen – this is the stage where hair is actively growing

Catagen – the end of the hair growth stage. This is a progressive rather than an abrupt process.

Telogen is the resting phase where the hair follicle is not making any new strands of hair.

A substance known as Transforming Growth Factor, TGF-B1, helps to end the active growth stage in the hair follicles affected by male pattern baldness.

Apigenin – a flavonoid – may slow this process down as it inhibits TGF-B1.

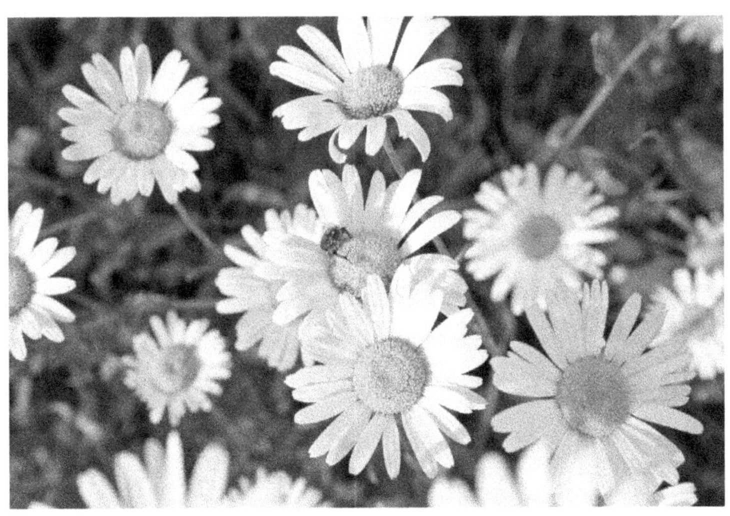

Curcumin – the active ingredient in turmeric – also acts to downregulate gene expression for TGF-B1.

This inhibition of TGF-B1 means that the ending of the growth phase is delayed or prevented.

I have often advised people that 'something that runs in the family' which is a genetic propensity does not mean that the condition will manifest itself in any individual with those troublesome genes. It is the epigenome which is the final decider of whether a condition occurs.   The epigenome is influenced by environmental factors so finding the key which turns on or off genes can make the difference. In male pattern baldness, apigenin may be the key that turns off the genes that bring the active growing state of hair to an end.

Now, apigenin is found in chamomile, parsley, celery, artichokes, spinach and oregano. The dried forms are particularly rich in apigenin.

As well as eating the above, there is nothing to stop you making an infusion of any of the above and applying this to your head for half an hour or so before washing it off.

Oregano and chamomile particularly are very easy to grow. Tiny amounts of oregano boiled up in water and allowed to cool will elicit tiny amounts of oil which has antibacterial properties.

The time taken up in making your own hair products is often much less than buying them from the supermarkets.

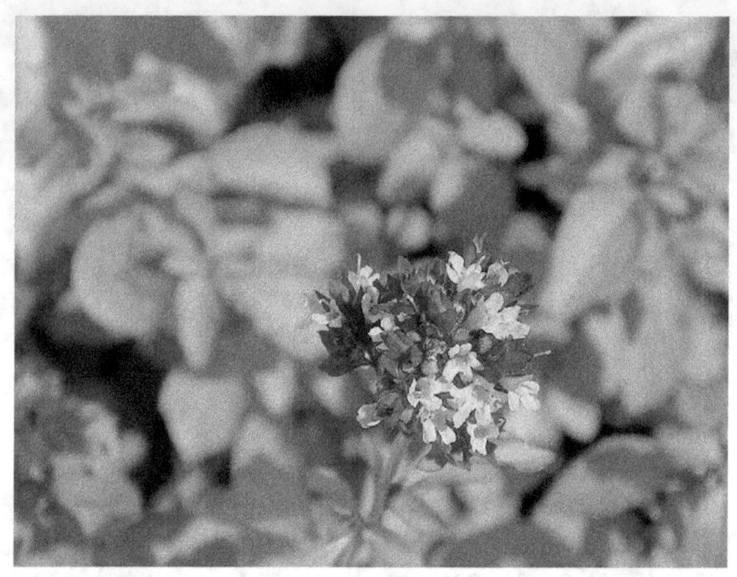

Oregano can spread rapidly in the garden but given its superb properties can be forgiven.

Another substance which is implicated in hair thinning and loss is DHT or dihydrotestosterone.

 DHT is an androgen male hormone and is responsible for male characteristics like deep voice but women do produce DHT too. However, the amount that they produce is far smaller.

For testosterone to be converted to DHT the enzyme 5-alpha reductase is required.

Testosterone+ 5-alpha reductase = DHT

Now before we go any further we need to know that DHT upregulates   the expression of TGF-B1 which we know stops the active growth of hair.

The process of hair loss now looks like something found in the diagram below.

How Hair Growth is Slowed or Ends

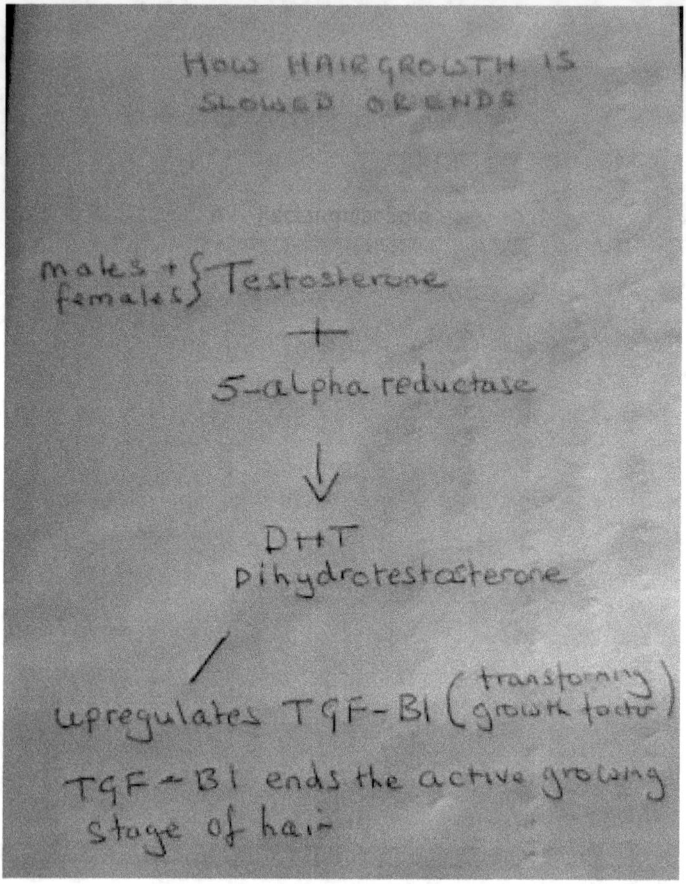

HOW HAIR GROWTH IS
SLOWED OR ENDS

males + females } Testosterone

+

5-alpha reductase

↓

DHT
Dihydrotestosterone

upregulates TGF-B1 (transforming growth factor)

TGF-B1 ends the active growing stage of hair

There are a number of reasons why hair loss occurs which impact some of the processes above.

Stress, for example, causes the stress hormone, cortisol to be released in high amounts. The hormone cortisol narrows the blood vessels carrying nutrients and oxygen to the hair follicles.

 In addition, not only is adrenaline increased but testosterone and DHT, too.

DHT binds itself to the androgen receptors found on the hair follicles. This results in what is known as miniaturisation of hair follicles which become progressively thinner. Women will, for example, find that their pony tail feels much thinner than it did when they were younger even though they may have the same number of strands.

Below you can see a picture of a non-healthy follicle bulb followed by a healthy follicle bulb.

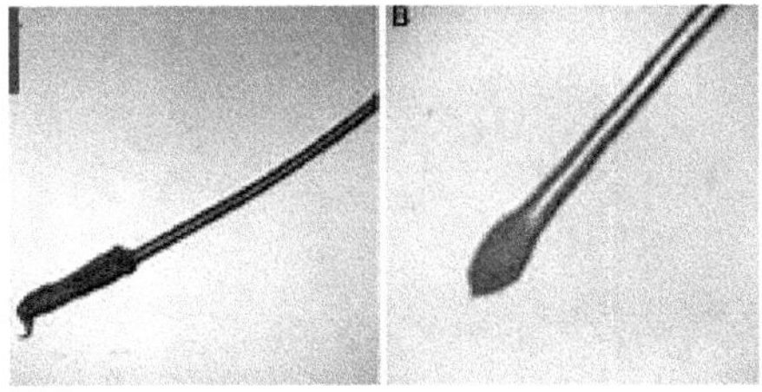

In addition to curcumin and apigenin, magnesium and rosemary oil are superb DHT blockers.

Ideally, magnesium should be in dietary form. it is found in soya beans, nuts, dried brewer's yeast, whole-wheat flour, bananas, green leafy vegetables, brown rice, dried peas, meat of all types, seafoods, dried fruit and many vegetables

It is difficult to see how magnesium deficiency occurs but magnesium deficiency is rife.

Deficiency symptoms are:

Painful swallowing

Weakness

Fatigue

Vertigo and convulsions

Muscle cramps and tremors

Nervousness

Nystagmus (involuntary eye movements)

Unsteadiness

Hyperactivity in children

Arrhythmias

Palpitations

Low blood sugar

The causes of magnesium are many and include:

Malnutrition – for example, due to anorexia nervosa

High dietary intake of calcium, vitamin D and saturated fats

Reduced absorption due to antacids, laxative abuse and diuretics

Kidney disease, diabetes, alcoholism, cancer, antibiotics, drugs used for cardiovascular disease

The contraceptive pill

High dietary milk intake

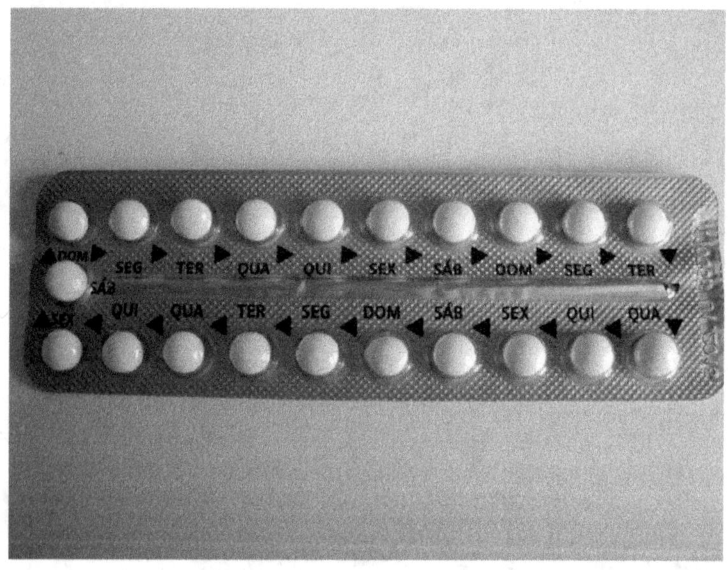

The contraceptive pill can cause a deficiency of   magnesium which can indirectly cause hair thinning and loss.

Rosemary oil is a wonderful oil which forms part of my hair regime.   It imparts a clean healthy smell, has anti-inflammatory and antimicrobial properties

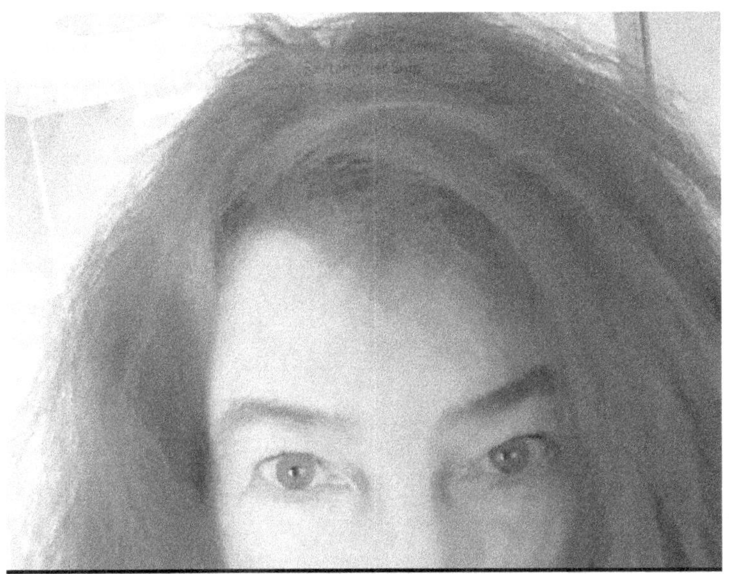

Hair care using rosemary oil – 70 years old in 2023

I merely massage a very small amount of rosemary oil into my scalp weekly. Leave it for half an hour and wash out. I will use a couple of drops rubbed into my palms to stroke over the top of hair to keep the shine.

That's it really as I do not have time to do anything else with my hair.

Of course it is helpful to try and address more than one area when trying to slow the progression/thinning of hair loss. We could do this by trying to reduce the impact of alpha-5 reductase so that it cannot convert testosterone to DHT.

There are a number of nutrients that will inhibit this conversion. By far the most effective are Reishi mushrooms which have 70-80% efficacy in inhibiting alpha-5 reductase.

In addition, saw palmetto and green tea have lesser, but still useful, efficacy.

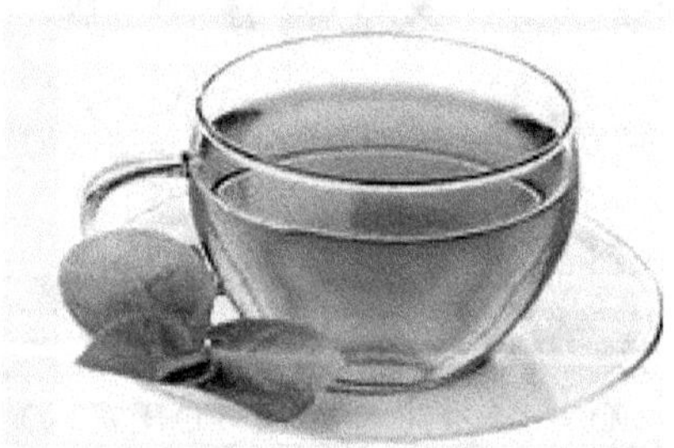

Green tea inhibits alpha-5 reductase which slows down hair thinning and loss.

MSM for hair growth

Hair is made up of a protein called keratin. By now you should know that proteins like keratin, are made up of amino acids. There are twenty-two amino acids some of which will combine to form specific proteins. For example, the protein that forms hair and the protein that forms skin are entirely different in composition but each performs a specific function based on its unique characteristics.

When the body makes keratin it needs four main amino acids for its synthesis. These are:

- cysteine

- lysine

- Arginine

- Methionine

Cysteine is the major player in helping to form keratin. It contains sulphur which improves hair texture, elasticity and strength. Cysteine is an essential amino acid which means that your body can't make it, itself and has to be taken in from the diet. Sulphur containing foods can be found in the allium family, such as onions and garlic, but egg yolks also contain sulphur as do seafood, organ meats and dairy produce.

Lysine is an essential amino acid which stimulates collagen production. It is also vital for healthy hair growth, helping to boost hair production. An essential amino acid means that it must be taken in through dietary means. It is found in similar foods to that of cysteine. However, it does not contain sulphur.

By far the best sources of lysine are meat, cheese, (especially parmesan) eggs, cod and sardines. Plant based foods are tofu and soy protein but because of the connection with thyroid cancer that soy foods have, I do not believe that these should be eaten any great quantity especially as the incidence of thyroid cancer is increasing and parallels the addition of soy based products to readiest meals.

Fenugreek seed also contains useful quantities of lysine.

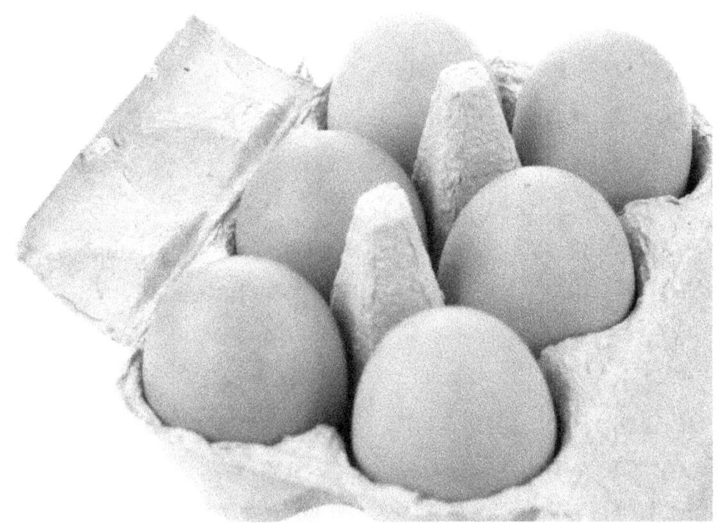

Eggs are a good source of lysine

Arginine is a conditionally essential amino acid which means your body does produce it. However, at times of injury or infection, you may need more dietary arginine than you are eating in your daily diet. Arginine is found in red meat, dairy products and nuts.

Arginine stimulates blood circulation around your hair follicles. It is a vasodilator so useful for lowering blood pressure. Cortisol, the stress hormone is a vasoconstrictor and is an unhealthy state for hair given that the narrowed blood vessels find it much harder to deliver the nutrients and oxygen that are also necessary for strong, healthy hair growth.

Methionine is the only other amino acid, besides cysteine which contains sulphur. It is an essential amino acid that helps to slow down the greying of hair.

MSM is a substance which is rich in organic sulphur which, as we've already learnt is a vital building block for healthy bones and connective tissue.

MSM is normally found in fresh raw food and meat. It is a white crystalline powder and can help treat diseases of older age such as osteoarthritis as well as help form healthy hair and skin. It contains a huge 34% of sulphur and, as such, can contribute to thick, healthy hair quickly.

MSM is quite bitter and not at all palatable so it may be better to find a MSM in capsule form.

Although we would expect good skin results in about four weeks - given that skin turnover is about one month - hair takes far longer to show the results of a diet which helps promote hair health.

MSM is found in a wide range of foods including Brussels sprouts, garlic, onions, leeks, legumes, wheat germ and green leafy vegetables like Kale.

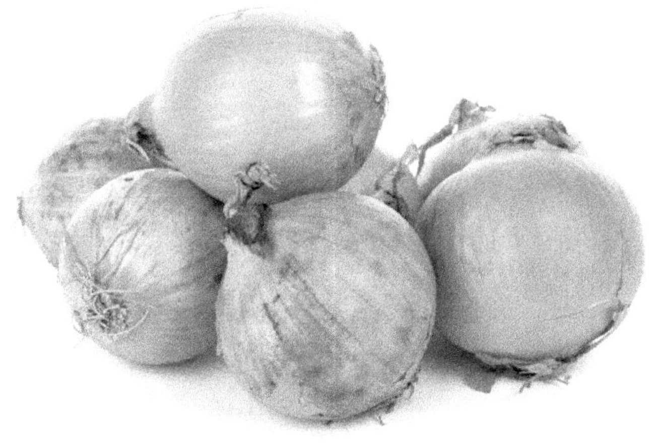

Onions contain MSM and contribute to hair health

Now, onions have long been known to help grow and strengthen hair. They are anti-inflammatory so help to keep the hair follicles healthy. It is not unknown for devotees of good hair health to massage onion juice into their scalp overnight before washing it out the following morning.

I love onions but prefer to eat them. Their versatility means that they can be eaten every day.

We cannot leave the subject of healthy hair without looking at the subject of the B complex and how they contribute to this complex process.

The B complex are a group of vitamins with similar properties. The first one discovered - B1 - is named thiamine, the second - B2- riboflavin. The final B vitamin – B12 – has great importance for cognitive function and a deficiency has symptoms similar to dementia. Some of the vitamins like inositol which used to be vitamin B8 are no longer considered to be 'vital' so have been reclassified and are not always added to supplements of the B complex. The benefits of the B complex are better tabulated below.

Vitamin	Benefits
Thiamine B1	Lowers blood vessel constriction and plays a vital role by converting nutrients into energy that the hair follicles can use.
Riboflavin B2	Helps to activate niacin and B6 which are necessary for healthy hair growth as well as having antioxidant capacity.
Niacin B3	Niacin stimulates hair growth increasing fullness
Pantothenic acid B5	Helps to nourish the hair follicle

Pyroxidone B6	It has a role in protein metabolism and makes sure that the hair cells have the amino acids needed to make hair proteins
B7 biotin	This vitamin stimulates keratin production.
B9 Folate/ folic acid	Helps to reduce greying, thickens and promotes growth

Good sources of the B complex are wholemeal foods, yeast based products, organ meats like liver and kidney, beans and nuts.

Healthy Bones

When we reach the age of about thirty we have reached peak bone mass. If we have always been very thin or done little weight bearing exercise. then it is quite likely that our bones are more fragile than we would like them to be.

Our bones, like our skin, contains collagen so if not enough bone and collagen forming foods have been eaten then, we are more at risk of osteoporosis, or fractures, as we age.

Interestingly, studies have shown that those who eat onions have a 20% less chance of osteoporosis than those who don't eat onions.

Onions have a number of benefits when it comes to bone health. They contain the essential amino acid cysteine which, as we have seen, is a major building block of collagen. Bone contains collagen. However, onions also contain boron.

Boron is a trace mineral. One of its functions is to assist other minerals and vitamins perform at their best.

As well as helping prevent osteoporosis, boron is associated with arthritis relief and increasing calcium and magnesium absorption which, in themselves, act as pain relief. Boron is a major player in helping your joints function as they should.

Boron is found in onions, tomatoes and apples but not as much as it used to be. Modern farming means that much of it has leached out of the soil. Boron deficient tomatoes look 'scabby' and have inward curling leaves when growing.

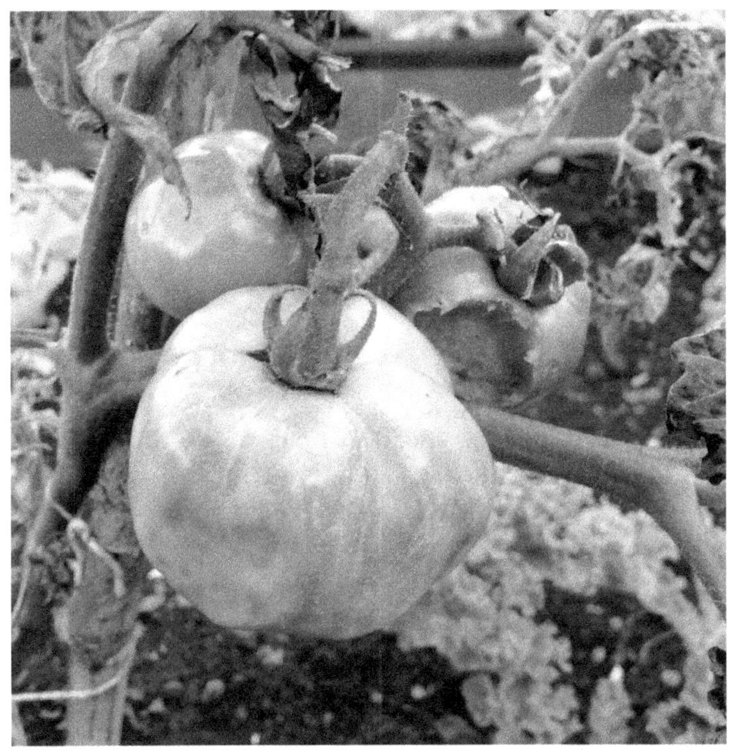

Boron deficient tomatoes

Apples may have brown spots in the flesh. Whatever way you look at them they do not look healthy.

Although we have already covered some of the benefits of vitamin D, it is also essential for bone formation as it helps calcium to enter the bones.

Calcium and magnesium are essential minerals for bone health and can be found in dairy foods and green leafy vegetables.

if you have read through the book thus far, you will see the recurring theme of 'green leafy vegetables.' They seem to be a panacea for all conditions especially as we age.

However, we cannot leave the subject of bone health to vitamin D, magnesium and calcium alone. Connective tissue is far more complex. Zinc, for example, is needed to accompany calcium into bone.

Is osteoporosis reversible without drugs? I have not come across any studies which promote that, as such, but there are plenty of studies which show that osteoporosis can be improved.

In order for this to happen we need to

- Perform strength/ weight bearing exercise

- Eat enough protein and perhaps consider taking collagen supplements

- Eat foods high in magnesium and calcium

- Eat foods high in boron. We need at least 3mg of this a day which is not easy to achieve.

- Take a vitamin D supplement of 2000IU's daily and get out in sunlight as much as possible.

- Take a diet which contains plenty of zinc. Zinc is an essential trace mineral required for the production of over 800 enzymes and macro minerals.

Seafood is particularly high in zinc.

Table showing essential nutrients for bone health

Boron	Found in apples and apple juice tomatoes, onions. 3mg required daily. Consider supplementation. Assists other major players in bone health do their job properly.
Calcium	Found in dairy foods, yogurt cheese, leafy vegetables, broccoli – required for strong bones – 800mg daily
Magnesium	Found in foods similar to that which calcium is found in. 800mg daily

Vitamin D	Vitamin D is found in sunlight, egg yolks, oily fish. It is required to allow calcium into bones. 2000 IU's required daily.
Collagen	Major structural component of bone. Bone broth is an excellent source.

Vitamin K is also becoming a major player in bone health. It has an important role in keeping calcium in the bones and out of arteries so it has added benefits for keeping the heart healthy.

Vitamin K is found in many dark green leafy vegetables and K2 is produced by bacteria in fermented foods.

K1 is needed to make the bone protein, osteocalcin. Osteocalcin contains the residues of the amino acid, glutamic acid. These bind to calcium. Vitamin K is essential for the formation of these residues.

The daily intake of vitamin K is 1000mcg. However, the average daily intake in the UK is approximately 100mcg. That is only a tenth of that which we require to keep our bones healthy.

Further, dietary K requires dietary fat for absorption. However, given the erroneous assumption that low fat diets are healthy, even the little we eat may not be absorbed.

A study found that those individuals with the highest vitamin K1 intake had a three-fold reduction in hip fracture risk.

Vitamin K2's benefits are that it is the most biologically active form and, as such, the most beneficial.

Vitamin K2 is produced by the fermenting of foods such as aged cheese, yogurt and kefir.

Osteoarthritis

Osteoarthritis is the commonest type of arthritis. About 50% of the population over the age of sixty years will suffer from this condition. It is a condition of older age and is generally, but not always, found in those over fifty years of age.

It is twice as common in women than it is in men and further, it is more prevalent in the white population than the black population.

Osteoarthritis is not considered to be an inflammatory disease. It occurs when the surface of the joint is damaged so that the smooth cartilage does not cushion the surface between the ends of the bones.

Cartilage is normally a shock absorber but can become worn and thin. This means the bone it is meant to protect becomes thicker. The process is slow and generally occurring in the weight bearing joints such as the hips and knees.

As the bone thickens bony outcrops grow into the joint membranes which usually become inflamed with synovial fluid. This can cause some swelling around the joint.

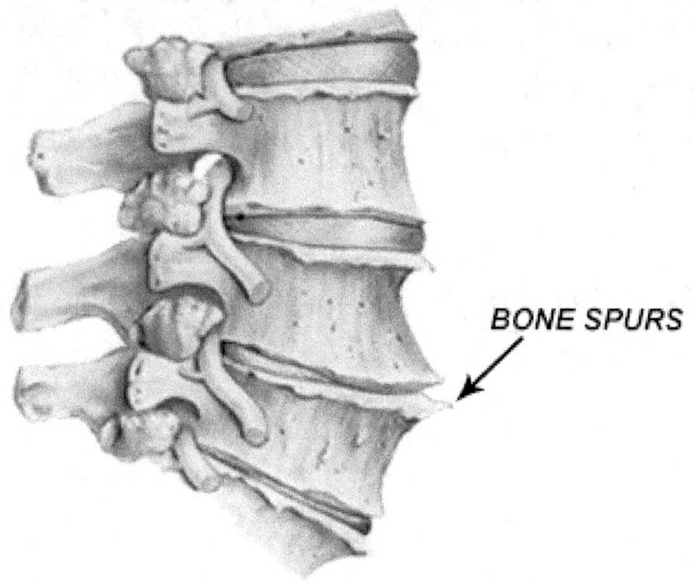

Bone spurs can occur anywhere and are   usually associated with wear and tear or injury.

The main symptoms are pain and stiffness with reduced joint movement.

Due to lack of use which is caused by the pain, muscle mass is lost. Treatments offered by a physiotherapist are designed so that muscle tone is built up.

Remedies for the pain for osteoarthritis.

Juniper berries

Sebastian Knapp was a 19th century priest and healer. He often prescribed juniper berries for a number of ailments. Juniper is able to cure rheumatism, skin disorders and gout. A little tipple of sloe gin would not go amiss and I know of a number of people for whom it works well.

Pectin and grape juice

This is another of those recipes which has been tried and tested by many with good results. Pectin and apple residue has been used in regenerative medicine in diseases such as osteoporosis, arthritis or osteoarthritis. Resveratrol found in red grapes has powerful anti-inflammatory effects so the above mix is a good treatment for osteoarthritis.

Certo is a proprietary pectin although you can make your own. We grow seven different varieties of apples. We cannot store 500 apples so we often make pectin from the skins and freeze it. We don't like to waste anything.

Just this afternoon I was talking to a gentleman who told me about the success he had for his arthritic knees after taking a tablespoon of cider vinegar every day.

I use apples in soup a lot. Apart from the fact that they contain boron, apples are a good base for soup. I also add them to casserole meats when they are cooking in the slow cooker, they thicken the gravy and produce a delicious gravy. There really aren't many dishes that you can't add apples to. They really are versatile. It is easy to see why the saying 'an apple a day keeps the doctor away' was coined.

Bone broths

I cannot praise enough the contribution of bone broths to the prevention and repair of cartilage.

Cartilage is difficult to repair. It is avascular which means that it does not have a blood supply. Most nutrients carried into cartilage do so by diffusion from the synovial fluid. This process is less effective as we age although keeping active certainly helps this process along. However, our eating habits and food preparation have changed and these also impact on our ability build up good cartilage.

One of the habits that we have dispensed with is boiling the bones up off joints of meat. This method involves long slow cooking and has largely been abandoned for the instant meal culture.

If I have a chicken, then I keep the carcase and throw it into the slow cooker with some onions and some apple peelings (I keep these in the freezer for such a time as this). The stock is then strained and can be used for soups, stews or risottos.

Bone broth is delicate and delicious and is one of the best medicines you can take for your joints.

I generally add some lemon juice to the cooking water as it helps the bones soften so that the nutrients leach into the broth.

MSM

Methylsulfonylmethane – which we have already discussed for its benefits for hair health, is a compound which has numerous benefits for relieving pain. Stiffness does not appear to respond as well to MSM, however.

MSM is found in fruits and vegetables but can also be obtained from health food stores as a powder which can be sprinkled over food if you can tolerate its bitterness.

Phenylalanine

Phenylalanine is an essential amino acid which has excellent pain relieving properties regardless of the cause of the pain. Thus it can respond to neuropathic and non-neuropathic pain, alike.   It is an adjunctive substance which means it can be used alongside your regular pain control and will enhance the pain relieving effect of it. It can be bought at any health food store as a powder. It has a slight taste - which is not unpleasant - and can be taken with water although it does not mix well.

Chondroitin Sulphate

Supplements for chondroitin sulfate are generally derived from animal cartilage. A study found that glucosamine and chondroitin were as effective for knee osteoarthritis as a well-known NSAID. Chondroitin sulphate is claimed to reduce pain and inflammation as well as improving joint cartilage.

Magnesium is an effective pain relief mineral and inhibits the breakdown of cartilage. Magnesium deficiency is quite common. A deficiency of magnesium is more likely to occur if the individual is using diuretics, laxatives or taking antacids like proton pump inhibitors.

Fibromyalgia. Soft tissue pain and the histamine connection

Fibromyalgia or fibromyalgia syndrome (FMS) is defined by the NHS as

A long term condition that causes pain all over the body. As well as widespread pain, people with fibromyalgia also have increased sensitivity to pain, fatigue (extreme tiredness) and muscle stiffness.

Common problems associated with fibromyalgia are

- Fatigue
- Pain and tender points
- Sleep problems
- Concentration and memory problems
- Headaches

- Anxiety and depression
- Morning stiffness
- Numbness and tingling in the hands, arms, feet and legs.

When we look at the symptoms that histamine can cause, they are not dissimilar. Further, histamine is a substance which can cause body wide pain and discomfort. We can discount prostaglandins as being a major player in widespread pain as prostaglandins tend to produce localised pain.

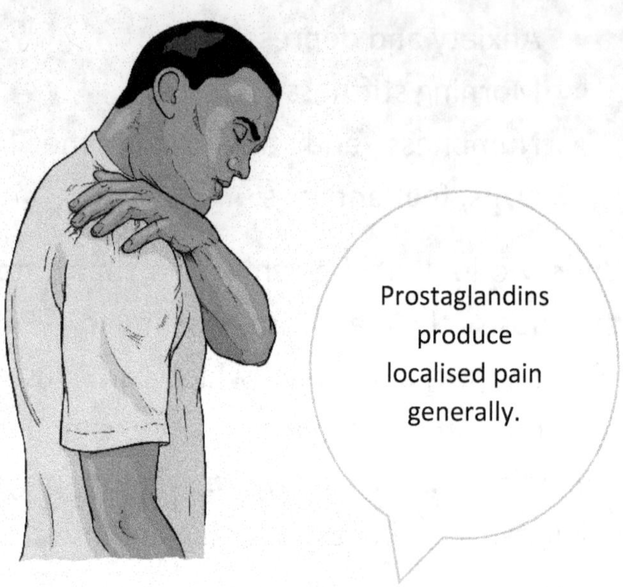

Fibromyalgia has a long history but has been renamed a number of times. It was originally known as fibrositis but 'itis' means inflammation and it did not appear as though there was any widespread inflammation involved in the condition.

In 1986 the antidepressants that raised brain levels of serotonin and/or nor-epinephrine were found to be effective in the treatment of fibromyalgia.

The drugs amitriptyline and doxepin were also subsequently found to have potent antihistaminic properties. This may have accounted for their pain relieving properties.

Over the counter antihistamines work very well on histamine intolerance and have very few short term side effects apart from a tendency to cause drowsiness. Some of the newer antihistamines are less likely to cause drowsiness.

However, antihistamines should not be taken long term. Histamine is needed for memory and recall. Long term use is associated with dementia.

 One of the unwanted side effects of antihistamines is that they have the potential to cause weight gain. This is thought to be due to the fact that histamine reduces appetite. Therefore, antihistamine can increase appetite.

Histamine has entered more and more foods in the food chain. Tomatoes and pickled foods contain lots of histamine. Fermented foods such as cheese and yogurt also contain histamine.

In 1963 yogurt was introduced by Ski to the UK for the first time. In many cases it has become a daily addition to the diet with it being a popular lunchtime snack. It is also added to Granola, eaten as a raita and eaten with fruit as a dessert.

As food intolerances rise, we need to look further than dairy which appears to be blamed. The increase, in recent years, in lactose intolerance is unusual since bovine milk, in its full fat glory, did not present a problem when there were not any alternatives.

Perhaps an alternative theory is that food intolerance may be due to the increase in foods containing histamine which sees yogurt and kefir as a major inclusion to the diet.

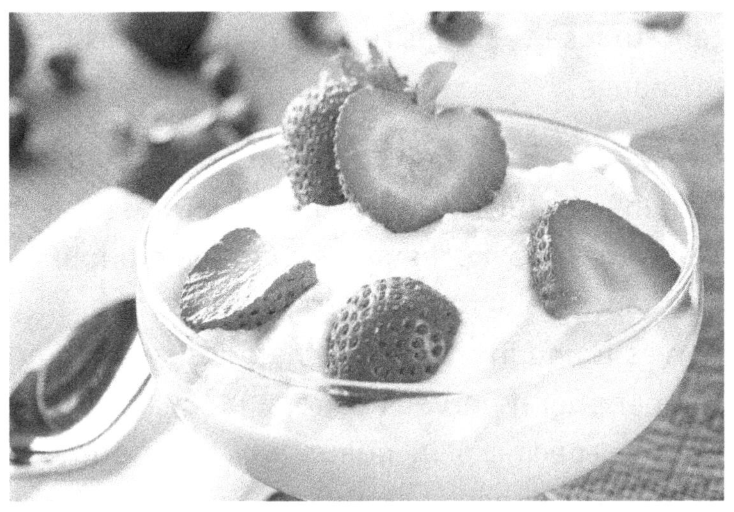

Indeed, sales of yogurt have risen by 40% since 2021 due to clever marketing promoting it as a health food.

Histamine, while a potential problem for those with a propensity to food intolerances or allergies has a beneficial impact on those with active sex lives. Histamine is required for orgasm to be reached as well as the strength of the orgasm. This effect is found in both males and females. As such, its impact may be useful for women going through the menopause who tend to lose their desire for sex during this time of change.

Substance P has also been implicated in fibromyalgia. It is one of the brain messengers believed to be dysregulated in this condition. As Substance P is released from specific sensory nerves found in the central nervous system and the peripheral nervous system, it could account for the specific pain points which sufferers of fibromyalgia have. However, it also causes widespread pain.

The treatment for excessive Substance P is different to that of histamine intolerance and it may be that treatment for both needs to be simultaneous for a couple of weeks. After that, the treatment for either excessive Substance P, or histamine intolerance, can be slowly withdrawn to see what the response is.

Finally, malic acid which is found in apples and pears, has also been found to reduce the pain of fibromyalgia and soft tissue injury.

Reluctant Bowels

Constipation is not one of those subjects which is given much of an airing unless it is in hushed tones or is the subject matter of comedy programme. We laugh and yet we are embarrassed. We would rather go to the GP with a cold, a bunion or an abscess. Our bowels are taboo and became so shortly after we were potty trained. We do not know what words we should use when trying to explain our discomfort and we have so few to describe the difficulties we might be having, anyway. Nevertheless, we have to give them the attention they are due for reluctant bowels and ageing appear to go hand in hand.

There are a number of definitions for constipation. These include 'unsatisfactory defaecation' which doesn't really mean anything as well as being quite hard to pronounce.

Another definition describes it as thus

Infrequent and frequently incomplete bowel movements. Constipation is the opposite of diarrhoea and is commonly caused by irritable bowel syndrome (IBS) diverticulosis and medications.

Medicine Net

Physicians tend to define constipation as the number of days between bowel movements while patients are more likely to describe their difficulties by describing the bowel movement. They may, for example, describe their stools as hard as golf balls or like rabbit pellets.

Constipation does cause serious distress and discomfort. It is not a minor complaint and in some cases be the cause of being admitted to hospital. In whatever way that you wish to look at it, constipation dramatically reduces the quality of life.

Fluids and fibre are supposed to be the cornerstone of preventing constipation but, in some cases, the addition of fibre can worsen the complaint, especially as we get older. Sometimes the reduction of fibre is the answer to a long standing problem so we will look at that in more detail. Are more fluids the answer? Not necessarily. It is still possible to be constipated while drinking adequate amounts of fluid.

Meanwhile, there are a huge number of medications which can cause this distressing complaint. These include diuretics, antacids and narcotics. Diuretics appear to be given more or less routinely to the elderly and cause a great many problems in the process. We shall explore the reasons for this later.

 Equally there are a huge number of medical conditions which can cause reluctant bowels. Most neurodegenerative disorders and an underactive thyroid are examples of these.

Constipation is not a condition in itself. It is a symptom of an underlying problem. A little investigation or a tweak to the diet can alleviate this problem in double quick time saving a lot of unnecessary tests and examinations.

Many old fashioned remedies work very well and we shall explore these in more detail and why they work. Prunes, for example contain a chemical called oxyphenisatin.   It is closely related to Bisacodyl, Sodium Picosulfate and Phenolphthalein.   Long term use of oxyphenisation was associated with liver damage and so it was withdrawn. More recent studies show that other compounds in prunes, including other phenolic compounds and sorbitol, are more likely to provide the laxative effect

Natural phenolic compounds do play a part in cancer prevention and treatment. Many phenolic compounds are to be found in herbs and include tannins, curuminoids, coumarins, quinones, flavonoids and lignans among others.

Sorbitol is a fruit-derived sugar. The body only metabolises it slowly. It is used in diet foods and is called a' nutritive sweetener.'   It has four calories in every gram and in that respect is similar to table sugar and starch.

It is used in diet foods or foods which are labelled 'sugar-free'. Nevertheless, it can raise blood sugar levels. It may be sugar free but it is not carbohydrate free.

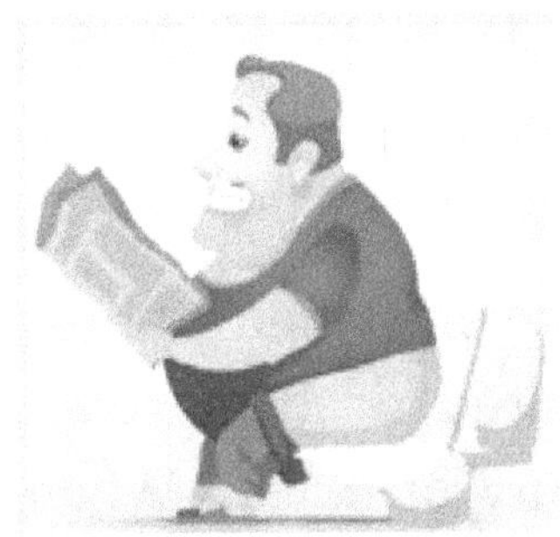

It should be emphasised that if anyone has concomitant weight loss with constipation that they should see their GP immediately. Any difficulties which are not alleviated, within two weeks, by the methods included in this book should serve as an indication that a visit to the GP should be booked for further exploration.

Causes of Gastroparesis

Gastroparesis is a digestive disorder that slows or stops the movement of food from the stomach to the intestine. It is generally a chronic disease and, as a result, may come and go. It is quite common in people with neurodegenerative disorders such as Parkinson's disease and multiple sclerosis as well as patients with diabetes mellitus.

Gastroparesis can develop when the vagus nerve's action is impaired or damaged by a nutrient deficiency, injury or illness. When the movement of food is slowed then the initial symptoms are abdominal pain and bloating.

At the upper end of the gastro intestinal tract, such delayed emptying may result in gastro-oesophageal reflux disorder but constipation is also one of the severe symptoms of gastroparesis.

Studies have shown that people with gastroparesis who have energy deficient diets are more likely to suffer from constipation.

Thiamine deficiency is quite common in the elderly and may contribute the problems mentioned. The deficiency may occur due to poor dietary habits, a lack of absorption – which is very common in the elderly – or the over consumption of thiamine inhibitors which include:

Tea

Coffee

Alcohol

High carbohydrate diets

Some medications, like the diabetic medication, Metformin, degrade thiamine rapidly.

Thiamine acts like a spark plug igniting glucose and oxygen to produce energy in the mitochondria, the powerhouse of every cell.

It enables the stomach cells to release acid without which the valve at the top of the stomach would not close leaking the stomach contents. The consequence of this is gastro - oesophageal disease, indigestion, heartburn.

The correct acidity also helps open the valve at the bottom of the stomach so that the contents are released into the small intestine. This prevents bloating and abdominal distension.

Further, thiamine is needed to make acetyl choline. Acetylcholine is a chemical messenger which acts in the central and peripheral nervous system on autonomic functions.

The autonomic nervous system is part of the peripheral nervous system and is involved in the bodily functions that we don't think about such as gut function.

In addition to thiamine, dietary choline is needed for the synthesis of acetylcholine. It appears that choline is deficient in most diets too so that the 440mg of choline for females and 550mg of choline for males is rarely reached. It is therefore of no surprise that delayed gut transit is a particularly common problem.

Choline is found in good amounts in organ meats, especially liver, eggs, fish, nuts and beans.

High fibre diets are not suitable for patients with delayed stomach emptying. The stomach normally empties its contents in a co-ordinated fashion into the small intestine but with gastroparesis muscle contractions are disorganised and the stomach empties too slowly.

Fibre delays gastric emptying. Further, it may clump together and form a bezoar.

A bezoar is a tightly packed mass of undigested or partially digested material which builds up in the digestive tract. It can cause a blockage. Bezoars are found in animals as well as humans and are most commonly found in the stomach.

Further down the intestinal tract, when the motor activity of the colon is compromised, it cannot propel the stool along the end of its journey. Normally the colon 'sleeps' when we sleep and there is little activity from it. On waking, the colon also wakes up. It begins its propulsive movements and these continue throughout the day. This will stimulate the bowel to evacuate.

The vagus nerve is the main nerve which controls the upper gut and the beginning of the large bowel. The colon is essential in helping to maintain an optimum amount of electrolytes and water. Electrolytes are body salts which regulate nerve function.[5]

An imbalance of electrolytes can easily disrupt gut motility. A number of medications can disrupt the electrolyte balance and these include medications such as diuretics and laxatives.

When potassium is lost – a side effect of these medications - then hypokalaemia can occur. Hypokalaemia is characterised by weakness and fatigue. The muscular weakness found in

---

[5] Common electrolytes are sodium, potassium, magnesium and chloride

hypokalaemia isn't just confined to skeletal muscle. It can affect smooth muscle and as such, be responsible for dyspnea,[6] abdominal distention and constipation. When the hypokalaemia is severe then rhabdomyolysis[7] may occur which is often accompanied by muscle cramps.

Unfortunately, increasing fluids – which is the most oft recommended advice – does not work to alleviate constipation in this case. The underlying cause is potassium loss and thus not fluid related. Increasing fluids only works on those who are constipated due to dehydration.

Increasing fibre will just aggravate constipation. If the bowel is not moving or moving only slowly then the fibrous meal will sit in the colon and become a hard solid mass.

The remedy for hypokalaemia is clear. Either the medication causing the condition must be withdrawn - or changed - or an increase in foods containing potassium must be eaten.

---

[6] Dyspnea - breathlessness
[7] Rhabdomyolysis – breakdown of muscle tissue

High potassium foods are bananas, oranges, melons, apricots, grapefruit, prunes, raisins, dates, cooked spinach, broccoli, potatoes, mushrooms, peas and cucumbers among many others.

Some people are naturally concerned that rebound constipation may occur if they give up laxatives since this appears to be a popular, but erroneous, belief. The Gastroparesis and Dysmotilities Association state that there is no evidence to support the belief that rebound constipation might occur after discontinuing laxatives. Further, the bowel does not develop a laxative dependency nor, despite possible misuse of laxatives, is there a potential for laxative addiction.

Hypomagnesia – low magnesium levels – is also a side effect of diuretics and can cause constipation. Both loop diuretics and thiazides are involved in excessive magnesium excretion. Nevertheless, other causes of hypomagnesia include poor diet. Individuals with disturbances in intestinal absorption may also suffer from poor magnesium absorption with subsequent constipation.

Magnesium draws water into the intestines. It works as an osmotic laxative and, this increase in water, stimulates bowel motility. It also helps to soften the stool, triggering a bowel movement and helping to make stools easier to pass.

Foods which are rich in magnesium include

- Meat
- Dairy products
- Fish
- Green leafy vegetables
- Wholegrain bread
- Brown rice
- Nuts
- Chocolate (however note that the iron in chocolate can dysregulate the bowel in some people).

A low fat diet is also recommended for gastroparesis as fat in the diet may delay gastric emptying. However, other studies show that a high fat diet increases gut motility[8]

The reasons given for increased gut motility due to a higher fat diet were that

- Some of the fat might pass through to the colon increasing its motility
- More bile acid is released which increases gut motility. However, take note that in order to synthesise enough bile acid, vitamin C is needed to convert cholesterol to bile acids.

From the above studies it appears that a high fat diet may delay gastric emptying and exacerbate gastro oesophageal reflux disease but may increase gut motility in the colon. As with any tweaks to the diet - in order to alleviate gastroparesis - it is trial and error as to which approach will suit any one individual.

---

[8] https://www.nature.com/articles/ejcn2010235

An interesting finding from the study, which is not common knowledge, is that the high fat diet reduced triglycerides, total cholesterol and low-density lipoprotein cholesterol while increasing high density lipoprotein cholesterol.

A diet low in fat and fibre is recommended for gastroparesis until correction of any thiamine or choline deficiency stirs the bowel into action. This may take up to 2 months to correct. Smooth pureed foods are also recommended which should be served as six small meals a day.

The thiamine regime will be given at the end of this book.

Although gastroparesis does occur in individuals with neurodegenerative disorders, the cause is more likely to be due to diuretic and laxative use which has disrupted the electrolyte balance.

In the elderly, who are very frequently prescribed diuretics, this should be the first consideration if they are complaining of constipation. Even the smallest dose of diuretic can cause problems. If a medication can act as a diuretic, even in   small doses, it has the ability to impact bowel motility as well.

Difficulties arise if the diuretic is not seen as contributing to the gastroparesis. It is not unusual to find that the sufferer will then be prescribed a laxative to deal with the diuretic induced constipation. The loss of electrolytes causes further harm not just to the gastro intestinal system but the central nervous and cardiovascular system.

Other medications which are associated with impaired gastric emptying are

- Narcotics
- Tricyclic antidepressants
- Calcium channel blockers
- Clonidine
- Dopamine agonists
- Lithium
- Nicotine

- progesterone

However, some smokers would argue that nicotine appears to increase gut motility. If this is the case then nicotine patches may help increase gut motility for some, if not all, individuals.

Human Growth Hormone and GABA

Most people have heard of Human Growth Hormone (HGH) but do not generally know what it is or what it does. This chapter will then give insight into a vitally important anti-ageing substance.

HGH is a hormone which is made in the pituitary gland. AS we age, the body's HGH levels decrease, which have led some scientists to believe that if we could raise HGH levels then this has the potential to reverse some of the effects of the ageing process. However, when HGH is taken by mouth it is destroyed in the acidic environment of the stomach. In order to benefit from HGH it has to bypass the stomach and be injected straight into the bloodstream.

It is possible to purchase injectable HGH online and some GP's may prescribe it off label.

However, this is not the easiest way to obtain HGH.

There are a lot of pills and potions that are sold which state either contain HGH or will help produce it in the body. Those containing HGH will not work given that they will be destroyed in the stomach and so it would be a waste of money to buy them in the first place.

A study showed that oral administration of an amino acid which is also an inhibitory neurotransmitter elevated resting serum growth hormone concentrations.

The purpose of the study[9] was to test the hypothesis that GABA ingestion stimulates immunoreactive GH (irGH) and immunofunctional GH(ifGH) release at rest.

Eleven resistance trained men (18-30 years) participated in this randomised, double blind,

---

9

https://www.ncbi.nlm.nih.gov/pubmed/180910 16

placebo-controlled, cross over study. During each experimental bout, participants ingested 3g of GABA or a placebo (P), followed either by resting or resistance exercise session. Fasting venous blood samples were taken at various intervals.

At rest the participants who'd had GABA were tested with those who had the placebo. The conclusions reached from the data were that ingested GABA elevates resting and post exercise irGH and ifGH concentrations but the extent to which it contributes to muscle growth is not known.

Now that we have shown that HGH can occur due to the ingestion of GABA, then it would be useful to know what we can expect if we take GABA supplements. These are:

- Loss of fat and muscle gain
- Increased energy levels
- Increased cardiac output
- Fewer wrinkles and improved skin elasticity
- Increased bone mass

- Increased memory retention
- Enhanced sexual appetite
- Improved sleep quality

GABA may also contribute to weight loss by its ability to induce restful sleep. A good night's sleep is associated with weight loss since this is when HGH is released. People who take GABA tend to lose weight quite effortlessly. As such increasing GABA can help those with middle age spread as there is loss of fat and muscle gain, the body becomes much more contoured too.

GABA is normally prescribed in doses of 200mg before bedtime to aid restful sleep. However, its fat burning capabilities, which are linked to the production of HGH, would require doses of approximately 3g on an empty stomach before bed. However, it is better to start at 1g - and work up in 500mg increments daily - until you find a dose which aids sleep. This dose would also promote weight loss.

In the UK, it has just become illegal to sell substances which promote HGH. This ban is indicative of the effectiveness of GABA in helping increase levels of HGH.

 However, GABA can be bought online. In addition, thiamine helps to increase GABA.

There aren't any foods which contain GABA. It is made from another amino acid, glutamine, which is found in animal protein such as meat, fish, eggs and cheese. Fermentation also aids GABA synthesis.

Studies have shown that when yogurt is eaten regularly, then weight loss occurs. This was thought to be due to the calcium content, However, as yogurt is a fermented product, it may have contributed to weight loss by a greater synthesis of the weight reducing GABA.

L-theanine – another amino acid - has been shown to increase GABA, serotonin and dopamine. It also helps to decrease cortisol.

 L-theanine is rapidly absorbed and results in reduced anxiety within a few minutes.

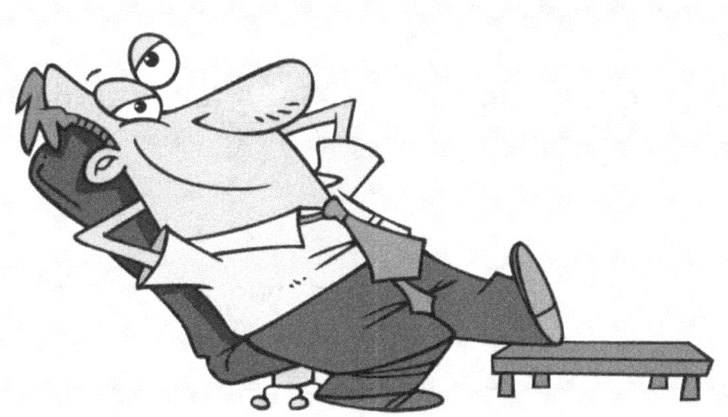

L-theanine results in reduced anxiety within minutes.

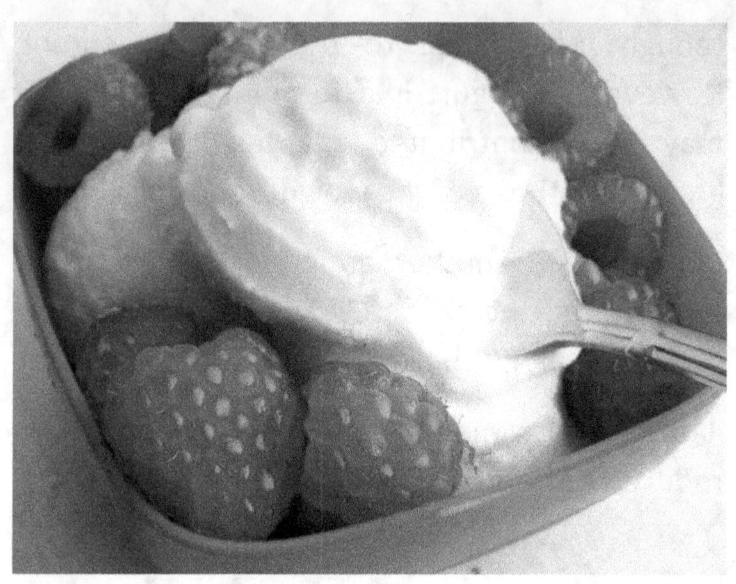

Yogurt can help increase GABA levels through its fermentation process

However, L-theanine has very few natural sources. It can be found in mushrooms and tea leaves. Most people reach for a cuppa when they need to wind down. That's the theanine effect. It makes sense to drink your tea strong so that you extract as much of this calming substance, from the leaves, as possible.

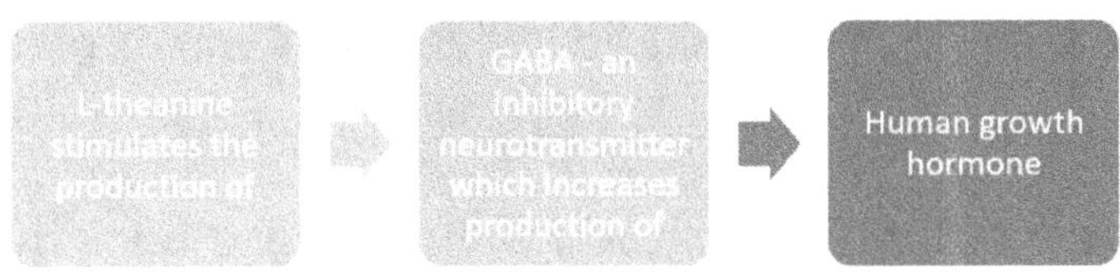

The concept of brewing the tea for three minutes has clear benefits. Leftover tea can be used in lots of ways. It was not unusual to soak dried fruit in cold tea before making the Christmas pudding.

Here is an iced green tea recipe for you to try.

Ingredients:

2 pints of water

4-6 green tea bags

One orange and one lemon sliced

Sweetening agent – honey, sugar, sweetener

Method

Place all the ingredients – apart from the fruit - in a jar with a fitted lid. Place in a warm place for 3-4 hours.

After this time add the fruit and place back in a warm place for a couple of hours.

Serve over ice after it has been sweetened further, to taste, if desired.

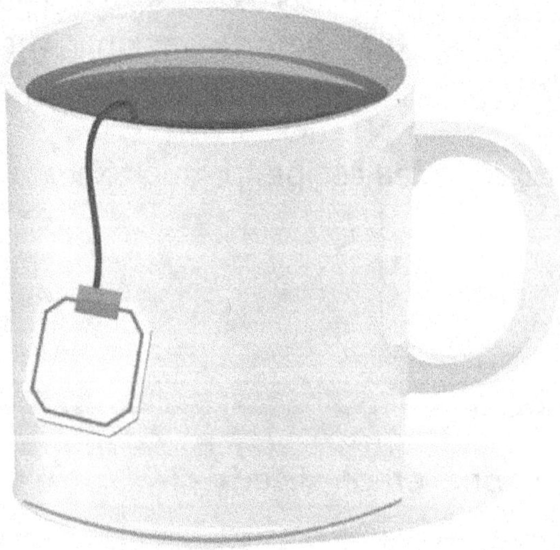

There is sound scientific reasoning why a cup of tea has 'pick me up' properties.

Taurine

Taurine and the immune system

The immune system is of special interest when we are looking at ageing. The ability of the immune system to cope with harmful stimuli such as damaged cells, cancer cells, pathogens and irritants diminishes as we age.

Acute inflammation is a response to harmful stimuli. It is our innate system that is responsible for generating inflammatory mediators such as histamine.

Inflammatory mediators, like histamine make blood vessels leaky This leakiness allows immune system cells, access to the damaged tissue.

The Japanese have a life expectancy that is among the highest in the world. The famous 'Island of Longevity' – Okinawa has the world's highest percentage of people who have lived to over 100 years old.'

The diets of these people contains a high intake of taurine.

Taurine is an aminosulphonic acid that is the most abundant free amino acid in humans. It plays important roles in the body such as:

- Maintenance of calcium homeostasis
- the regulation of fluid within cells (osmoregulation)
- membrane stabilisation
- promotes cardiovascular health
- hearing function (helps prevent or improve tinnitus)
- electrolyte balance
- insulin sensitivity
- heart failure

Taurine also plays a role in acute inflammation that is associated with oxidative stress. In addition, it has antimicrobial effects. Taurine and its association with longevity are so convincing that taurine has become known as the

'Nutritional factor for the longevity of the Japanese'.

Acute inflammation is a physiological response of tissues to harmful stimuli such as pathogens, damaged cells or cancer cells and irritants. This response, mediated predominantly by innate immunity, is responsible for the elimination of injurious stimuli and the subsequent healing process.

 As we age our bodies cannot produce an optimal amount of taurine. Further, it is likely that vegetarians and vegans will not have adequate amounts of taurine since these diets lack taurine. Additionally, disease states such as cancers, kidney and liver disease generally lack sufficient taurine.

Taurine is beneficial in neurological and metabolic conditions.

Animal models have also shown that taurine supplementation lowers blood pressure by attenuating nerve impulses in the brain that drive blood pressure up.

Moreover, taurine helps to reduce the signs of atherosclerosis by reducing arterial thickness and stiffening.

Taurine and eye health

Taurine is well known for its protective effects on eye health. Optimum levels help prevent age-related vision loss. It has especial use in diseases of the retina where oxidative stress can lead to such conditions as. macular degeneration. Normally, there is plenty of taurine to be found in the retina, but, of course, the concentrations decrease with age. Taurine helps to maintain levels of nerve growth factor that is required for preserving the health of the retina.

Taurine and seizures

Taurine, has the ability to reduce or eliminate seizures, too. It can do this by binding to GABA receptors which are the chemical messengers that have a calming influence on the brain. Taurine helps the brain from firing in an uncoordinated fashion which produces seizures.

Taurine and hearing loss

 Taurine has been found, in some cases, to be able to reverse hearing loss as well as eliminate tinnitus associated noises. The hair cells in the ear are dependent on the flow of calcium in and out of the cell. When calcium flow is restored to normal then hearing is also restored as taurine helps to maintain normal calcium influx into auditory cells

The normal diet produces about 59mg of taurine. The human body requires about 3g or 3000mg so unless we eat a lot of fish or muscle meat or organ meat like liver and kidney then we are likely to be deficient in this substance.

Taurine is available online or in health food shops in powder, capsule and tablet form. It is normally recommended that 3g is taken daily. This is equivalent to 3000mg.

Antioxidants

These are substances that can prevent or slow down damage to cells caused by free radicals.

Free radicals, also known as reactive oxygen species, are unstable molecules that are produced by the body. They are the result of processes that the body undergoes, such as inflammation and stress. They also occur as a result of environmental stress in the form of cigarette smoke, sun exposure or pollution such as car exhaust fumes. If the free radicals cannot be removed quickly enough then oxidative damage occurs. Oxidative damage is linked to a large number of diverse diseases that include:

- Motor neuron disease
- Parkinson's disease
- Alzheimer's disease
- Respiratory disease
- Cancer
- Arthritis
- Stroke
- Any chronic inflammatory disease

Antioxidants are sometimes called 'free radical scavengers.' They help to neutralise free radicals in our body. The body makes some of its own antioxidants but many antioxidants come from plants. They are then referred to as 'phytonutrients'. The body, however, cannot make its own antioxidants without the ingestion of correct nutritional substances.

Many antioxidants are found in fresh fruit and vegetables. Vitamin C, however, is easily destroyed by sunlight, cooking methods and storage.

Different foods provide different antioxidants. Brazil nuts, for example, provide selenium. Selenium helps:

- Reduce hair loss
- Certain cancers
- Relieve asthma symptoms
- Protect against cardiovascular disease
- Prevent mental decline

A study[10] argued that the human body is in a constant battle to keep itself from aging. Research[11] suggests that free radical damage to cells leads to the pathological changes associated with ageing.

Studies[12] have shown that coffee drinkers — coffee is full of antioxidants - are less likely to get ALS, Parkinson's disease and Alzheimer's disease. These are all diseases of advancing age.

 In a study[3] of elderly mice with Alzheimer's disease, for example, caffeine was found to reverse cognitive impairment as well as lower brain amyloid-beta levels.

In an animal model of ALS, coffee was found to increase antioxidant enzyme capacity in the

---

[10] https://www.ncbi.nlm.nih.gov/pmc/articles/PMC3249911/

[11] Ashok BT, Ali R. The aging paradox: Free radical theory of aging. Exp Gerontol. 1999; 34:293–303.

[12] https://academic.oup.com/aje/article/174/9/1002/168671

brain of male G39A mice, improving motor performance as a result.

A caffeine derivative, known as LM11A-24 appears to protect degenerating motor neurons.[13]

Coffee contains a number of important antioxidants as well as vitamin B3.

Science Direct[14] states that:

Coffee beans are a rich source of biologically active compounds such as caffeine, chlorogenic acids, nicotinic acid, trigonelline, cafestol, and kahweol, which have significant potential as antioxidants.

It is worth exploring these antioxidants a little further.

Chlorogenic acids

These have a wide array of benefits including having an anti-inflammatory effect in the brain.

---

[13] https://www.ncbi.nlm.nih.gov/pubmed/17004921

[14] https://www.sciencedirect.com/science/article/pii/B97801240473 89000039

They also help to reduce the incidence of type 2 diabetes and may have benefits for heart disease.

Trigonelline

This substance has many potential benefits.[15] It is neuroprotective, anti-migraine and reduces neuron excitability which is implicated in neurodegeneration. Further benefits include:

- Lowers blood fats
- Lowers blood sugars
- Improves memory
- Antibacterial
- Antiviral
- Anti-tumour
- Reduces diabetic auditory neuropathy
- Reduces platelet aggregation

---

[15]

https://www.researchgate.net/publication/225288518_Trigonelline_A_Plant_Alkaloid_with_Therapeutic_Potential_for_Diabetes_and_Central_Nervous_System_Disease

Cafestol and kahweol

Both of these substances tend to impact positively on the liver lowering inflammation in this organ. There are studies that link liver and gut activity with Alzheimer's disease. The brain is intricately connected to all other organs.

Final thoughts

I hear lots of people state, 'There's nowt (nothing) to being old. Equally, I hear just as many people say, I've been to the doctor and they say there is nothing that can be done as it is just old age.'

I cannot agree with either of those two statements even though I understand where people are coming from when they say that.

Older age does not have to be full of aches and pains, stiffness, obesity, wrinkles and poor eyesight. It should be a time of freedom when the fetters of working life are not tying you down; when you have the freedom to do things that you enjoy doing.

If you have bone pain and arthritis, take boron. If you are anxious increase L-theanine. If you lack sleep, take GABA enhancing foods. In short, learn to doctor yourself so that you can enjoy life with all the fullness that it is meant to have.

Ageing should have no more challenges than any other time in your life.

Additional information, protocols for health conditions

The thiamine regime

300mg of thiamine

300mg magnesium

A good vitamin B complex

Take for 3 months then have a 6 week break then continue but lower thiamine to 100mg daily.

This regime will help sleep, pain, gastrointestinal disorders, cardiovascular and central nervous system disorders.

Protocol for viral and bacterial infection

It would be true to say that vaccinations do not hold the answer to the prevention of viral or bacterial infections. Quite simply, if you do not have a robust immune system to begin with then any immune response will fail. If you do have a strong immune system, then you simply do not need   any form of external help

Viral and bacterial respiratory infection

The protocol for the above is given but can be used for other infections to good effect. The reasons for the protocol are given alongside the therapeutic doses and names of each supplement.

- Vitamin D3 20,000 IU's daily with a little fat for three days and then continue with 4000 IU's thereafter
- Quercetin (found in apple juice and onions)
- Vitamin C – 6-8g daily until the infection is cleared
- Zinc- 25-50mg daily
- Allicin 200mg once daily
- Cholesterol (as it neutralises bacterial toxins so in order to aid recovery, cholesterol lowering drugs should not be taken).

Further advice on the above protocol

1) **Vitamin D3 20,000 IU's daily** until the infection begins to dissipate. **Up to 50,000 can be given for one week in severe cases.** After the infection begins to subside, the dose can be reduced to the Recommended Daily Intake (RDI) of 4,000 IU's daily.

Between the hours of April and to the end of September, it may not be necessary to take vitamin D if you have been in the sun for more than 20 minutes a day.

Vitamin D is a fat soluble vitamin and cannot be absorbed without being taken with a little fat. Some full fat milk or half a slice of well-buttered toast is adequate.

Vitamin D activates the innate immune system which is the general defence immunity we have from birth. Some of the general defences we have are mucous membranes which prevent penetration of infective agents into our body, acidity on the skin which kills infective agents but which soap washing and hand cleansers destroy, general all-purpose immune system cells, among many others

Activation of the general immune system- which tends to keep most infective agents at bay – is necessary to activate the acquired immune system which has more specialist artillery at its disposal to deal with infective agents. However, please note that if you do not have adequate amounts of vitamin D in the first place, neither arms of the immune system can be activated.

Vitamin D produces its own Antimicrobial peptide (AMP) which is known as Cathelicidin. This is a broad spectrum antimicrobial which is effective against many other infective agents such as fungal infections in addition to bacterial and viral infection.

2) **Zinc 25mg to 75mg for one week**. If using the higher amount, then use 75mg for only 3 days and then reduce to 25mg.

Zinc is essential for the synthesis of approximately 800 macromolecules many of which are involved in defence against infection. Zinc prevents viral spike protein from attaching and entering cells. It tends to be more effective with small amounts of quercetin.   If too much zinc is taken, then nausea will ensue and you must cut back.

3) **Quercetin. 100mg daily.** Quercetin is a B type flavone that is anti-inflammatory in nature and works alongside zinc in preventing infection.   Onion or leek soup has plenty of quercetin in it and could be a consideration for light meals during convalescence instead of a quercetin supplement which is quite bulky.

4) **Vitamin C 2000mg rising to 6000-8000mg should bacterial infections such as pneumonia be present.** Vitamin C has anti-inflammatory properties at lower doses and is rapidly used up at times of infection and stress. At higher doses it acts therapeutically in the same way that antibiotics do.   There are no reason why

even higher doses cannot be
administered until bowel tolerance is
reached (faecal contents will be watery
and explosive at this point) where this will
evidence that all tissues are saturated
with vitamin C.

Vitamin C is generally fine on the stomach but if
you have a tender stomach there are forms
which are less acid. These tend to be more
expensive and are generally not required.

**Other useful natural substances to address
infection**

**Allicin 450mg daily but 200mg is the standard
dose.** The active ingredient in garlic, it has
efficacy against gram positive and gram

negative bacteria and enhances antimicrobial activity in the lungs.

It passes through cell membranes and reacts with circulatory glutathione. Research is not clear whether it develops sufficient concentration in tissue to exert the desired clinical effect but it is effective in the vapour phase so is useful in a nebuliser.

Cholesterol – adequate cholesterol is vital for the health of the respiratory system. People on cholesterol lowering drugs are at a distinct disadvantage when overcoming respiratory infection. Cholesterol is required for the synthesis of the cell membrane of every cell including immune system cells. Research has shown that those on cholesterol lowering drugs are more likely to die from respiratory and gastrointestinal infection. Cholesterol is needed to neutralise bacterial toxins which destroy tissue in order to spread through it. Specifically, the neutralisation of the gram negative bacterial lipopolysaccharide (LPS) is importance since LPS is a pro typical trigger for sepsis

Protocol for cancers

The amino acid blend to assist in your immune system function is found below.

These amino acids are all freeform acids

All the immune system fighter such as T cell, antibodies and white blood cells are primarily composed of strings of amino acids which are used to synthesise the enzymes vital to targeting and destroying cancers.

The amino acids need to be blended together in specific parts.

These are:

Arginine – 9 parts

Glutamic acid – 10 parts

Cysteine 0.5 parts

Glycine 3.5 parts

Cofactors for the above are:

Vitamin A, vitamin B complex, vitamin C and vitamin D3

Calcium

Magnesium

Selenium

The amino acid blend is taken at 10mg dosages 3 x daily.

For infection with H pylori

- Take one tablespoon of virgin olive oil with 200mg of allicin twice daily
- 300mg thiamine and 300mg magnesium and a vitamin B complex for one month then re-evaluate

For stomach ulceration

- Glutamine as advised on package
- Riboflavin 100mg
- Vitamin C 1g three times daily

Tinnitus

3g of taurine in divided doses daily

4000 IU's of vitamin D daily taken with a little fat

Magnesium 200-300mg daily

25mg zinc daily

Indigestion and avoiding the PPI's

The dangers of the Proton Pump Inhibitors (PPI's) like Omeprazole and Lansoprazole are immense.   PPI's were developed in the 1980s. PPI's were, of course, prescribed to address problems like GERD and indigestion.   Omeprazole, which appears to be most commonly prescribed   PPI, commenced its introduction to the commonly prescribed medications in 1988. Although, other PPI's have since been developed, they are generally benzimidazole derivatives.

PPI's work by inhibiting gastric cells from pumping acid into the stomach. This is the opposite action to the diverse and vital actions of vitamin B1, which is known to impact every cell in the body. Indeed, vitamin B1 - also known as thiamine - is implicated in dry, wet and gastrointestinal beriberi which can damage major organ systems.   In the latter, it is partly the lack of gastric acid that causes major injury to the systems of the body.

Stomach acid serves a number of purposes. The low pH – optimum stomach acid has a pH of 2 - kills of any infective agents which may pass down into the stomach. Optimum stomach acid also   breaks down food so that it can be digested more easily. Vitamin B12, for example, cannot be separated from its protein source if stomach acidity has decreased. It is a common problem with the elderly who are particularly prone to vitamin B12 deficiency, especially as the symptoms include, among others, dementia. Moreover, without sufficient stomach acidity, the valves in the stomach cannot work, so the upper valve cannot close keeping stomach acid where it should be – in the stomach. Further, the lower valve which leads into the small intestine, cannot open so contents have nowhere to go. The partly digested food ferments causing bloating and distension.

It is not just   the absorption of vitamin B12 that PPI's affect either. Some of the vital major nutrients such as calcium, magnesium, zinc, the B vitamins are all affected. The impact of deficiencies of any – never mind all of these – can be life changing, reducing the quality and quantity of life.

Zinc is involved in   the synthesis of over 800 macromolecules and enzymes, the lack of which any would be a risk factor for a specific condition. Zinc is required to accompany calcium into the bones Lack of zinc, as well as calcium, will result in fragile bones and a significantly increased risk of fractures. Calcium reduces seizure risk and taken little and often, reduces chronic pain. Calcium is also used in indigestion medications as it is antacid in nature but does not prevent the gastric cells from releasing acid into the stomach when needed.

 Zinc is needed to provide viruses from entering host cells and the replication of virus. People with leg ulcers tend to have lower amounts of zinc in their system which zinc supplementation addresses. Zinc also protects the stomach and is useful in cases of indigestion.   Eye and skin lesions are common in zinc deficiency as is hair loss.

Vitamins are called vitamins because they are vital to the working of the body. The B complex are well known for their positive impact on energy levels and   mood disorders. The B complex are depleted   rapidly at times of stress. Therapeutic amounts of the B complex call alleviate depression, anxiety and psychosis as just some of the mood disorders they can address without the side effects of prescribed medications.

How then, do we address the problems which may arise and which may lead a sufferer of GERD to be given PPI's? PPI's are given, for example, for those who are on steroids or NSAID's such as Naproxen in order for the latter to control pain and inflammation. In some people they may cause gastritis or ulcers so PPI's are given to try and address this. However, they tend to throw up more problems than the reason why they were prescribed in the first place.

I am not in favour of masking symptoms without attempting to address the underlying cause so that may be an area which takes much time but that time should be given in order to prescribe appropriate treatment. Therefore, where pain and inflammation occur, I would be addressing that but certainly not by reducing the absorption of calcium, magnesium, zinc and the B complex, all of which prevent damage to the stomach lining! Vitamin C, although an acid in its form ascorbic acid, helps to heal the stomach lining and can be used instead of PPI's to prevent damage to the stomach lining. After all the pH of ascorbic acid is not as acidic as stomach acid is itself. Should problems occur then vitamin C ascorbate is the gentler buffered form of vitamin C.

Vitamin   B3 – niacin - may cause gastritis in some susceptible people. This does not appear to be a problem in naturally derived sources of vitamin B3 but many have reported that the added vitamins in fortified foods do cause all sorts of digestive problems including indigestion. This particular fortification of food with niacin was intended to avoid pellagra, the symptoms of which include, dementia and diarrhoea and thus, may be specifically relevant to the elderly.

In order to control stomach acidity there has to be an understanding that the acidity is vital for the functioning of the gastrointestinal system and that it is not the acidity that is wrong, it is the leakage of the stomach contents which is of concern. In order to improve that you would have to help the gastric cells release acid which can only be actioned if sufficient thiamine (B1) is available. As we have seen thiamine absorption is disrupted when PPI's are taken.

We have two further handy weapons when it comes to addressing conditions like GERD. These are two amino acids – arginine and glycine – which address the problems of acid leakage and oesophageal lesions well.

Studies have shown that when oesophageal lesions were addressed by the administration of dose dependent L-arginine and glycine that the buffering action was found to offer significant protection.

However, the amino acids L-alanine and L-glutamine were found to produce a deleterious effect on the oesophagitis

Is it then that as diets change that de novo conditions arise giving opportunity for pharmaceutical companies to encroach into this area, producing new medications which address problems that would be addressed by simple changes in diet. As a medical nutritionist, I firmly believe so. De novo conditions arise due to environmental factors   which are introduced in a subtle way. We accept them because if we do become aware of them we are informed by those in 'authority' that they are good for us. I find nothing good about the PPI's. Their impact is negative and long lasting. They do not address the underlying issue and, as such, the recommended 'Do not take for more than 8 weeks' may continue for years; this often without any follow up from the GP.

Table showing the sources of L-arginine, Glycine, L-alanine and L-glutamine

Amino Acid	Sources
L-arginine (non-essential amino acid but those with certain conditions or elderly may need to supplement	Fish, red meat, poultry whole grains, beans and dairy products
Glycine (5g daily required) a Non-essential amino acid which can be made endogenously provided all the component contributors are supplied in the diet.	Red meat: (1.5 to 2 g per 100 g serving) Seeds (1.5 to 3.4 g per 100 g) Turkey (1.8 g per 100 g) Chicken (1.75 g per 100 g) Pork (1.7 g per 100 g) Peanuts (1.6 g per 100 g) Canned salmon (1.4g per 100g)
L-alanine – a non-essential amino acid.	Game and veal , protein powders – generally found in products intended to help with body building
L-glutamine	Eggs: 4.4% (0.6 g per 100 g of eggs) Beef: 4.8% (1.2 g per 100 g of beef) Skim milk: 8.1% (0.3 g per 100 g of milk) Tofu: 9.1% (0.6 g per 100 g of tofu) White rice: 11.1% (0.3 g per 100 g of rice) Corn: 1

Thank you for purchasing this book. Every time a book is purchased, a donation is made to one of the charities I am currently supporting. These can be found on my author's website. See below.

Other Health Related Books by the Author

- **The Reluctant Bowel**
- **A Weighty Issue**
- **Sleep, Perchance to Dream**
- **The Journey: EDS and chronic pain**
- **The MND diet: using nutrition to slow down the progress of neurodegeneration**
- **A Necessary Sorrow**
- **Pain: its causes and what can be done about it**
- **Pain: causes and treatment of pain associated with fibromyalgia, arthritis and soft tissue injury**
- **Effective treatment for stress, depression and anxiety**
- **Parkinson's disease: Dietary changes that work**

https://www.amazon.co.uk/~/e/B07BPQZ5CD